T0197290

# Where There Is No Child Psychiatrist

## A Mental Healthcare Manual

**VALSAMMA EAPEN** PhD FRCPsych FRANZCP
*Professor & Chair, Infant, Child and Adolescent Psychiatry, University of New South Wales, Sydney, Australia*

**PHILIP GRAHAM** FRCP FRCPsych
*Emeritus Professor of Child Psychiatry, Institute of Child Health, London, UK*

**SHOBA SRINATH** MD DPM
*Professor & Head of Child and Adolescent Psychiatry, National Institute of Mental Health and Neurosciences, Bangalore, India*

Illustrations by Kiriko Kubo
*London and Tokyo*

RCPsych Publications

# CAMBRIDGE
## UNIVERSITY PRESS

University Printing House, Cambridge CB2 8BS, United Kingdom

One Liberty Plaza, 20th Floor, New York, NY 10006, USA

477 Williamstown Road, Port Melbourne, VIC 3207, Australia

314-321, 3rd Floor, Plot 3, Splendor Forum, Jasola District Centre, New Delhi - 110025, India

103 Penang Road, #05-06/07, Visioncrest Commercial, Singapore 238467

Cambridge University Press is part of the University of Cambridge.

It furthers the University's mission by disseminating knowledge in the pursuit of education, learning and research at the highest international levels of excellence.

www.cambridge.org
Information on this title: www.cambridge.org/9781908020482

© The Royal College of Psychiatrists 2012

RCPsych Publications is an imprint of the Royal College of Psychiatrists,
17 Belgrave Square, London SW1X 8PG
http://www.rcpsych.ac.uk

All rights reserved. No part of this book may be reprinted or reproduced or utilised in any form or by any electronic, mechanical, or other means, now known or hereafter invented, including photocopying and recording, or in any information storage or retrieval system, without permission in writing from the publishers.

This publication is in copyright. Subject to statutory exception and to the provisions of relevant collective licensing agreements, no reproduction of any part may take place without the written permission of Cambridge University Press.

*A catalogue record for this publication is available from the British Library*

ISBN 978-1-908-02048-2 Hardback

Cambridge University Press has no responsibility for the persistence or accuracy of URLs for external or third-party internet websites referred to in this publication, and does not guarantee that any content on such websites is, or will remain, accurate or appropriate.

The views presented in this book do not necessarily reflect those of the Royal College of Psychiatrists, and the publishers are not responsible for any error of omission or fact.

The Royal College of Psychiatrists is a charity registered in England and Wales (228636) and in Scotland (SC038369).

# Contents

# Preface

This manual is a guide to the assessment and management of children and adolescents with developmental, behavioural and emotional problems. It has been written mainly for primary care professionals, especially primary care physicians and nurses, working in low- and middle-income countries. Most of these do not have specialist paediatricians or mental health specialists available for advice and further care. We believe it is important for these primary care health professionals to be better able to help children and adolescents with mental health problems than they can at the present time. We hope the manual will also be found useful by teachers, social workers and school counsellors, and other professionals working with children and adolescents in similar places.

# Acknowledgements

We would particularly like to thank Kiriko Kubo, who has provided such attractive illustrations, and Paul Carter, consultant community paediatrician, who has commented in detail on all the paediatric sections in early draft form.

We would also like to thank, as well as six anonymous reviewers, the following who have commented on the outline of the book and/or on different sections in draft form:

Lynne Boulter
Gerald Dingley
Paul Eunson
Tejas Golar
Elizabeth Goodburn
Hilary Heine
Elizabeth KE
Vibha Krishnamurthy
Anula Nikapota
Vikram Patel
Hernamali Perera
Jacob Roy
Diyanath Samarasinghe
Koyeli Sengupta
Henal Shah
Tony Waterston
Pat Wright

# Abbreviations

| | |
|---|---|
| ADHD | attention-deficit hyperactivity disorder |
| ASD | autism spectrum disorder |
| BMI | body mass index |
| CBT | cognitive–behavioural therapy |
| LAMI | low- and middle-income |
| PTSD | post-traumatic stress disorder |
| WHO | World Health Organization |

# List of tables and boxes

# CHAPTER 1

# Introduction

## 1.1 Mental health problems in children and adolescents

What do we mean by mental health problem? The term mental health problem covers a wide range of difficulties:

- it involves the mind rather than the body
- it can be mild, moderate or severe when it causes serious disruption to the lives of the child and parents
- it is common for children to show more than one problem
- it usually has more than one cause
- it can often be assessed and managed effectively by primary healthcare professionals.

## 1.2 Types of mental health problems

The following are different types of mental health problem. Each of these is described in more detail later on in the manual.

- Delays and deviations from normal development
- Habit problems in the early years, especially feeding, sleeping difficulties, bed-wetting and soiling
- Emotional problems, especially anxiety and depression
- Behaviour problems, including extreme disobedience, temper tantrums, aggressive behaviour, stealing, lying, truancy and attention-deficit hyperactivity disorder (ADHD)
- Self-harm
- Mental health difficulties arising from chronic physical illnesses
- Physical symptoms for which no physical illness is found
- Severe mental disorders, especially psychoses
- Alcohol and drug dependency
- Stressful or damaging experiences, especially child abuse
- Having more than one of the above problems, which is very common.

## 1.3 Importance of mental health problems

Many studies of mental health problems have now been carried out in low- and middle-income (LAMI) countries. They all show that children in these countries, including, for example, India, China, the United Arab Emirates, Colombia and the Philippines, have either the same or higher rates of mental health problems than children in high-income countries.

Between 1 in 5 and 1 in 10 children have mental health problems that reduce the quality of their lives at any one time.

Children with these problems are frequently seen in primary healthcare clinics, but they are often not identified by those working in such clinics. One study carried out in four LAMI countries showed that nearly 4 out of 5 children who attended clinics with mental health problems were not recognised to have such problems by the health professionals who saw them (Giel *et al*, 1981).

Methods that could be used by health professionals working in primary care are available that would result in effective assessment and management of such cases. We shall describe these methods later in the manual.

Health professionals receive very little, if any, training in this area of work. There can be no real substitute for personal supervision of clinical work in this area, but we hope that this manual will play at least a small part in informing primary healthcare professionals about these problems and give them some idea as to how they might be assessed and managed.

## 1.4 Main causes of mental health problems in childhood

There are three main reasons why children and adolescents develop mental health problems: genetic influences, their physical health and stresses in the environment, especially within the family and at school.

1   Our genes influence the type of temperament we have.
2   The physical health of children affects the way they feel and behave. Both acute and chronic illness can have important influences on children's mental health.
3   Stressful experiences at home and at school may be upsetting for children. Children who face stress may also learn from such experiences so that they are better able to cope with them in the future.

Commonly there is an interaction between these three factors. In particular, the way children respond to stress depends at least to some degree on their genetic make-up. Some children are built to withstand even severe stress; others become sad, anxious or angry when faced with relatively minor stress.

The amount of influence that genes have varies with the type of problem that a child shows. In children who show attention and concentration problems and cannot sit still, genes are very important, but the way parents bring their children up is less so, although, of course, parents do have some influence. But, for example, in children who are aggressive, lie or steal, genes play a much smaller part. In such children, it is aspects of the family environment such as the way parents behave and the amount of antisocial behaviour in the neighbourhood and at school that matter. Genes and stress interact in complicated ways.

**Case 1.1**
Lalitha, a 15-year-old girl, is brought to the clinic with period pains by her mother, but it is soon revealed that this is a minor problem. The main difficulty is that she is crying all the time and feels life is not worth living. She was going out with a much older man, but he has now rejected her as he is already married. Lalitha has never shown any signs of depression previously – her mother says she was always a cheerful, happy, fun-loving girl. The health professional knows that Lalitha's mother has had severe depressive episodes, sometimes following quite minor stress. The health professional wonders whether Lalitha would have felt so depressed if she had not inherited some 'depressive genes' from her mother. Quite possibly if she had not been vulnerable to depression, Lalitha would not have reacted so badly. Now the health professional is worried that Lalitha's emotional problem might be too much

for her mother to cope with and that she too will become depressed. That, in turn, would make life more difficult for Lalitha.

Some people think that if a problem is caused by genes there is nothing that can be done about it. That is not true – sometimes one can help more with a problem that has a strong genetic influence than with one where parental behaviour is more important.

In fact, in deciding what to do, the health professional should not worry about how much of Lalitha's distress is influenced by genes and how much by the stress she has suffered. He will try to fit the appropriate care to Lalitha's unique situation and he will almost certainly be able to help considerably.

The main stresses acting on children are:

- disturbed family relationships, for example unhappy parental marriages, especially if accompanied by domestic violence
- loss by separation or death of family members, friends or pets
- physical or mental illness in parents, brothers, sisters or other family members
- alcohol or drug problems in parents
- problems in school (e.g. learning difficulties, bullying by other children)
- problems in the neighbourhood (e.g. gangs, high levels of violence).

Poverty in itself does not lead to mental health problems, but when money is very tight, parents often become stressed and worried and this can put severe pressure on children's lives. Subnutrition, closely linked to poverty, causes disturbances in a child's ability to learn by making them irritable, listless and hampering their development generally.

Man-made disasters such as civil conflicts and natural disasters such as earthquakes, tsunamis, floods and drought often result in families being split up, with children orphaned or separated from their parents. Situations with such high levels of stress involved are likely to lead to high rates of mental health problems.

# CHAPTER 2

# Assessment and treatment: general principles

## 2.1 Assessment

When carrying out an assessment, try to make the room in which you will see children as child-friendly as possible. The room may well be used to see adult patients as well, but if possible make sure that there is a chair that a younger child can feel comfortable sitting on. Try to make pencils and paper available. It is also helpful to have about three jigsaws for children of different ages. These are really useful for assessing the developmental age of a child. It is also helpful to have available about three children's books set at different levels. This will make it possible for you to do a rough check on a child's reading age.

You will not have a great deal of time to make an assessment, but assessing a child for a mental health problem will not be all that time-consuming if you know the right questions to ask (see below). Further, if you spend time at the beginning finding out about a mental health or development problem, you may save time later on. Children who have physical symptoms not due to physical illness may take up a great deal of time until you sort out what their problems are really about.

First, ask the mother an opening question, such as 'What is the problem?' Often you will have a good idea of the nature of the problem if you allow her to talk for as long as she wishes. Allow the mother to tell her story without interruption.

Do not miss the opportunity the assessment provides for observing the child and seeing his reaction to what the mother is saying. If he is more than 2 or 3 years old, try to bring him into the conversation. Observe the quality of the relationship between the child and his mother. For example, is she worried about talking in front of him if she is describing difficult behaviour or is she pleased to be able to tell you what a terrible boy he is? If you have been able to provide pencils and paper, take an interest in what he has drawn and praise him even if you think it is not at the level the child should be performing at at his age.

While you are listening to the mother and observing the child, keep in your mind that the main aim of the assessment is to provide information that will enable you to make some helpful suggestions. This does not necessarily involve making a diagnosis. In fact, a diagnosis such as 'depression' or 'conduct disorder' is not nearly as helpful as a summary and action plan that you can make when you have finished your assessment (see Chapter 3).

Make sure you have enough time to communicate to the mother at the end of the consultation how you see the problem. Check on how your summary matches with how she sees it. She and the child should feel encouraged and supported when they leave, not humiliated or more confused than when they first met you.

With some mental health problems it will be necessary to carry out a physical examination of the child (discussed throughout the manual where appropriate).

## 2.2 Taking into account local culture

The health professional needs to understand the language, beliefs/values and style of life of the members of the families he is trying to help. This is important in many different ways.

### 2.2.1 Language

The language used to describe mental health problems will depend on the country, city, town or village in which the health professional is working. In most places there is no word for depression as an illness. People can talk about sadness and misery, but not think of these emotions as becoming illnesses even if they are severe. We have already used the word 'adolescent' several times, but in some societies this word does not exist. Children grow into young adults without a transition phase in between. Local languages are likely to be rich in words that really matter to the people who use them, such as words for different types of crop or weather, but lack words for ideas that, until recently, they have had no need for.

### 2.2.2 Families

Multigenerational families (families in which grandparents, parents, sometimes uncles and aunts, and children all live together under one roof) are more common in LAMI countries than in high-income countries. This is important both in understanding mental health problems and in working out how children with mental health problems can be helped. For example, grandparents, especially grandmothers, often play a major role in bringing up children and, if this is the case, need to be involved in any proposed changes.

### 2.2.3 The way parents bring their children up

The health professional needs to know what is regarded as normal parental behaviour. For example, in some societies, parents who beat their children with a stick when they are disobedient are regarded as cruel and inhumane. In other societies, parents who do not use a stick to beat disobedient children are thought of as bad parents who do not mind how their children behave. Particularly when deciding whether a child has been physically abused, health professionals need to know what local people think of as normal. This does not mean that primary healthcare professionals should approve of normal practices when they know they are harmful. For example, there is evidence that children who are beaten by their parents are more likely to become aggressive and/or unduly anxious later in life even in societies where it is normal for parents to behave in this way (Gershoff *et al*, 2010).

### 2.2.4 Lifestyle

Knowing about what is regarded as normal lifestyle is vital for health professionals. In some societies, for example, a 16-year-old girl who wears make-up and goes out with boys is regarded as normal, whereas in other societies such behaviour would be thought of as completely outrageous and irreligious.

### 2.2.5 Different ways of showing distress

If there is no language or very limited language to describe distress, then people, including children, are likely to show how upset they are by developing physical symptoms. For example, a child who is really upset about the loss of a friend might not be able to talk about her feelings but might develop crippling headaches. In that way she would get sympathy and perhaps physical affection from her parents that she might otherwise miss out on. She might also be taken to a health professional, who needs to understand that although headaches are sometimes caused by brain disease, they are more likely to arise from emotional upset.

### 2.2.6 Beliefs about the cause of illness

In Western countries, physical illness is thought to arise from something going wrong in the body. That is true for all societies, but in some the matter does not end there. Why should the body be affected in this way? In some cultures all events are thought to have a supernatural cause and nothing happens by chance. In these instances, people are likely to believe that the person afflicted with illness has had a spell cast upon them, or have in some way upset the gods. Before health professionals tell parents what they think is the matter with their children, they need to know what the parents believe the matter is and why their child has been affected.

### 2.2.7 Beliefs about treatment

In some societies, the treatments for mental health problems that Western societies would regard as appropriate for children and adolescents are not seen to be at all useful. Instead, parents may go to a local healer, who may be a spiritual healer, witch doctor, *shaman* or priest. If parents have faith in such local healers, then provided they are not using harmful remedies, children may obtain as much benefit from them as they would do from Western-trained health professionals. Sometimes Western-trained health professionals are only consulted when the local healer has failed to produce satisfactory results. Such health professionals benefit from knowing about the alternative sources of help available to parents and, if possible, working with local healers rather than in opposition to them.

### 2.2.8 A cultural complication

Many health professionals work in localities where there are a number of different cultural groups, each with their own set of beliefs, attitudes and values. If they are to provide a comprehensive service, it is important that they are able to understand these differences and how they affect the lives of children.

## 2.3 Treatment

Decisions about how to treat a child with a mental health or developmental problem should follow assessment. Treatment is guided by the understanding of the problem that has been gained during the assessment, and the type of treatment that can be offered will depend on the skills of health professionals and the resources available to them.

Before offering treatment it is important that you find out what the parents have already tried. It can be frustrating if, after suggesting ways of helping a child, the parents then tell you that they have already tried all the measures you have suggested without any benefit.

Apart from relaxation exercises for anxiety states and tension headaches, there are basically two main types of intervention that can be used in dealing with mental health problems in children and families – listening and talking treatments and medication. These will be described in more detail in relation to the problems to which they can be applied. What follows is a brief general outline.

## 2.3.1 Helping through listening and talking

### Stress reduction

Sometimes it is clear that the child's symptoms are a response to stress. You can try to work out with the parents and child how this might be reduced. The stress may be within the family, at school or in the neighbourhood. An example might be suggesting to the mother that she is firmer and more consistent in her discipline. This might result in a reduction in the number of stressful arguments as the child no longer feels he can 'get away' with disobedience. Another example might be reducing the pressure on the child caused by examinations. What you are trying to do by using use this approach is make the environment (the world the child lives in) more friendly to the child.

### Cognitive–behavioural therapy

The idea behind this form of treatment is that children with problems often have a false set of thoughts or beliefs about the world and people around them. These false ideas affect their emotions, making them sad, anxious or perhaps angry. Thus fearful children have an exaggerated idea about the dangers facing them. Children with depression may feel that no one likes them when that is not the case. If one can successfully combat these beliefs, the child's emotional problems are likely to diminish or even disappear altogether. This reality testing approach will be discussed in more detail in the sections dealing with particular types of mental health problem. It has been found to be the measure most likely to produce changes of behaviour or emotional state. It should be combined with approaches that result in an increase in understanding of why children and parents are behaving in the way they are.

### Behaviour therapy

In this approach an attempt is made to change behaviour directly without dealing with underlying thoughts or feelings. This form of therapy is based on the idea that if one wants to change behaviour, one needs to know what happens both before and after the behaviour occurs. Both of these affect the likelihood of the behaviour occurring. For example, suppose a health professional is dealing with a child who constantly seeks attention. She might discover that the boy's attention-seeking behaviour only occurs when his sister is getting all the attention. She might also discover that the boy's attention-seeking behaviour always succeeded in stopping his parents giving his sister attention. A behaviour therapy approach would not try to find out why he is so attention-seeking. Instead, one would try and see what would happen if his sister were to be given less attention when her brother was around, and perhaps more attention at other times. Further, one could try and make sure that when the child was naughty, he got less rather than more attention, perhaps by sending him out of the room. As will be clear from later sections, most behavioural approaches stress the need to reward good behaviour rather than to punish unwanted behaviour.

### Improving relationships

The cause of problems some children experience lies in the unhappy relationships they have, especially with other family members. Using this approach, an attempt is made to help both children and other family members understand how things look from another person's perspective. Family members often need to be helped in this way to be able to show the love and care they really wish to show to each other. If it is possible, sometimes it may be helpful to arrange to see all the family members together (family therapy) to allow them to express their feelings about the referral problem. This often results in the family members realising that the problem does not lie in the child about whom the complaint is made, but more widely within family relationships.

### Parenting education

Although children receive a great deal of education on other subjects in school, they are usually not taught anything at all that will be of help to them when they take on the most important job they will have in life – the upbringing of their own children. Parents can be helped to improve the way they provide love and discipline, resulting in reduced behaviour and emotional difficulties shown by their children (see Chapter 15). This approach is of great importance in helping parents of children with developmental delay and in preventing behaviour problems.

### Increasing understanding

This is the main aim of listening and talking treatments, usually called counselling or psychotherapy. The idea is to help parents and children understand better the reasons why they are behaving the way they do. It usually involves helping them to look at what has happened in the past, so that they become more aware of how this is affecting what is happening now. This type of intervention has a good chance of making children and parents feel understood, but less chance of changing behaviour than the other forms of talking treatment described above.

## 2.3.2 Medication

Many health professionals provide medication at the end of a patient's visit. Further, many parents expect health professionals to prescribe or suggest medication and are disappointed if they are sent away without it. This makes life difficult, for although there is definitely a place for medication in the treatment of emotional and behaviour problems, most children who come to clinics would not benefit from it. They are likely to be helped by one or other of the listening and talking treatments described above.

However, parents and children sometimes find listening and talking treatments hard to accept and health professionals often do not feel they have the necessary skills to provide them. In this manual we try to help professionals to feel more confident in withholding medication when it is really not required. We also try to provide some basic skills in using listening and talking treatments in the relevant sections.

# CHAPTER 3

# Making a summary and action plan

This is a very short chapter but it contains information that will be important for the children and families that you see.

When you have finished your assessment and considered the treatment possibilities that are available, you will need to make a summary and a plan of action. This is sometimes called a formulation. Ideally, this is written down, but often lack of time will mean this is not possible. You should, all the same, make a summary in your mind of all the relevant information you have gathered and of the action you have decided to take.

## 3.1. Making a summary

You first need to decide whether the lives of the child and/or family members are being affected by the problem. Is the child's functioning at home or at school impaired by the problem? If the child is eating and sleeping well, getting on reasonably well with other family members, making progress at school and has friends whom he enjoys seeing, then there probably is no reason for concern. The mother may all the same have anxieties about the child and may well need reassurance, perhaps repeated reassurance, but the child does not need treatment.

If, however, the lives of the child and/or family members are being affected by the child's developmental progress, behaviour or emotional life, then you do need to make a summary and action plan. You need to include in your summary the following.

- The nature and extent of the problem or problems (often more than one of these is present):
    - developmental or intellectual
    - habit disorders
    - emotional disorders
    - behaviour problems
    - self-harm
    - mental health difficulties arising from chronic physical illness or disability
    - physical symptoms without physical cause
    - severe mental disorders, especially psychoses
    - drug use disorders, alcohol and drug dependency.
- The possible causes of the problems or problems:
    - genetic
    - physical
    - stresses arising from the environment (from the world in which the child is currently living), especially within the family or at school:

    a   traumatic or damaging experiences that have happened to the child in the past

    b   an interaction between any or all of the aforementioned possible causes. This is easily the most common situation.

Next, from your knowledge of the problem and of the possible causes in this particular child, try to understand how the problem has arisen, what is maintaining it, and what is most likely to help.

### 3.1.1 Example of a summary

**Case 3.1**

Raghu is an 8-year-old boy who has been suffering from headaches for 6 months. Having heard his mother's story and examined him, it is extremely unlikely there is a physical cause for his headaches. They do not sound like migraine. There are no obvious stresses at home or at school but he is under terrible pressure to do as well as his 10-year-old sister. He is probably not quite as bright as she is. It is likely that the headaches are stress-related and that the situation could be helped by making his parents more aware of the reasons he is experiencing them.

## 3.2 Example of an action plan

Raghu can probably best be helped by:

- a talk with his mother about the way some children experience pain when they are stressed and that some stress happens when children feel that their parents are disappointed in them
- asking him whether he feels he is not doing as well as his sister at school even though he is trying very hard
- asking his mother whether she thinks it is possible that he is comparing himself with his bright sister
- asking his mother and father to help Raghu to understand that they are really pleased with him, even though he is not doing as well as his sister
- activities that either his mother or father could do with him that he really likes and which are not stressful for him.

If at all possible, check on the effect of your intervention. If your intervention has not been effective, reconsider your summary and action plan and consider trying to help in other ways.

# CHAPTER 4

# Development and developmental problems

Children's development occurs along a number of different pathways.

- Gross motor: using large groups of muscles to sit, stand, walk, run, etc., keeping balance, and changing positions.
- Fine motor: using hands to be able to eat, draw, dress, play, write, etc.
- Language: speaking, using body language and gestures, communicating and understanding what others say.
- Cognitive: thinking skills, including learning, understanding, problem-solving, reasoning, and remembering.
- Social: interacting with others, having relationships with family, friends and teachers, cooperating and responding to the feelings of others.

Children develop along these pathways at different rates. The great majority develop normally, eventually becoming adults able to work and lead fulfilled social lives. Some children, however, have specific developmental delays or disorders, and a minority develop slowly in all aspects of their development. These children are said to have intellectual disability. Some children with mild or moderate intellectual disability, will either be partly dependent on others or will be able to lead lives that are normal in most respects. A small minority are affected with severe intellectual disability and will remain dependent on others throughout their lives.

In this chapter we will discuss:

- how to assess development in the early years of life, giving details of the 'milestones' that children achieve and pass during their development
- specific developmental problems:
  - language delay
  - stammering
  - reading difficulties
  - clumsiness
- autism spectrum disorder (ASD): delay and disorder in multiple areas of development.

For each of the above we will discuss the way the problems present, their likely causes, how to assess them, and how to provide help. We will discuss intellectual disability, previously called mental retardation, in Chapter 5.

## 4.1 Assessment of developmental delay

Developmental delay is a term used to describe children who are slow to develop in the first 5 years of life. It is usually children of this age who are brought to a health professional by their mother because of a worry that development is not normal. Such children need careful assessment. There are four possible outcomes to an assessment of development.

1    The health professional may identify that the child's development is within the normal range, and once the mother is reassured that this is the case, all is well.
2    The child's development is within the normal range but the mother is not reassured when you explain that this is the case. There is a problem that needs attention.
3    The child's development is somewhat delayed in one or more areas of development so as to cause concern. There may or may not be progress over time to bring the child within the normal range.
4    The child's development is definitely outside the normal range in most or all areas of development.

When conducting an assessment to see whether a child's development is a cause for concern, the following guidelines may be helpful.

•    Although you will wish as far as possible to observe the level of the child's development yourself, sometimes the most useful information comes from the mother. When in doubt, ask the mother whether the child can do a particular task. She will know better than anyone.
•    Try to get the mother to show you what the child can do rather than assessing the child without the mother's cooperation. Young children are very likely to cry and not show you what they can do if you take them away from their mother to carry out a task.
•    It is important to find out whether the child is generally slow to develop (global developmental delay) or whether the delay is limited to one or two areas of development (specific delay in development), as described on p. 11.

## 4.1.1 Developmental milestones

These are a set of skills or tasks that most children can do by a certain age. The following are guides to what most children are doing at particular ages. If they are not, this is likely to be a cause for concern. If the child is nearly performing the task at the expected age, this is obviously much less worrying than if the child is only performing like a child half their age. Mothers will want to know whether their child is going to 'be normal', or whether they will have to catch up. It is difficult or even impossible to give a clear answer to this question until the child reaches the age of 4 or 5 years. Children who by 18 months or 2 years are only at a level equal to half their age are likely to have some degree of intellectual disability as they grow up (see Chapter 5).

**At 3 months of age, is the child able to:**
*Motor skills*
•    Lift head and chest when lying on stomach
•    Follow a moving object or person with the eyes
•    Just able to grasp rattle when placed in hand
•    Wriggle and kick with arms and legs

*Sensory and thinking skills*
•    Turn towards the sound of a human voice
•    Respond to you shaking a rattle or bell

*Language and social skills*
•    Make cooing, gurgling sounds
•    Smile when smiled at

- Communicate hunger, fear, discomfort (through crying or facial expression)
- React to 'peek-a-boo' games

## By 6 months of age, is the child able to:

*Motor skills*
- Hold head steady when sitting with your help
- Reach for and grasp objects
- Move toys from one hand to another
- Pull up to a sitting position on their own if you grasp the hands
- Sit with only a little support
- Roll over

*Sensory and thinking skills*
- Open mouth for the spoon
- Imitate familiar actions you perform

*Language and social skills*
- Babble, making almost sing-song sounds
- Know familiar faces
- Laugh and squeal with delight

## By 12 months of age, is the child able to:

*Motor skills*
- Drink from a cup with help
- Feed self finger food such as rice or bread crumbs
- Grasp small objects by using the thumb and index or forefinger
- Sit well without support
- Crawl on hands and knees
- Pull self to stand or take steps holding onto furniture
- Stand alone momentarily
- Walk with one hand held

*Sensory and thinking skills*
- Copy sounds and actions you make
- Try to accomplish simple goals (seeing and then crawling to a toy)
- Look for an object, such as a spoon, that has fallen out of sight

*Language and social skills*
- Babble, but it sometimes 'sounds like' talking
- Say at least one word
- Show affection to familiar adults
- Show mild to severe anxiety at separation from parent
- Show fear of strangers
- Raise arms when wanting to be picked up
- Understand simple commands

## By 18 months of age, is the child able to:

*Motor skills*
- Pull, push and drop things
- Scribble with crayons
- Walk without help

*Sensory and thinking skills*
- Look for objects that are out of sight
- Follow simple one-step directions
- Solve problems by trial and error

*Language and social skills*
- Say eight to ten words you can understand
- Look at a person who is talking to them
- Ask for something by pointing or by using one word
- Direct another's attention to an object or action
- Become anxious when separated from parent(s)

## By 2 years of age, is the child able to:
*Motor skills*
- Feed self with a spoon
- Wash hands with help
- Walk up steps with help

*Sensory and thinking skills*
- Take things apart
- Explore surroundings
- Point to five or six parts of a doll when asked

*Language and social skills*
- Use two- to three-word sentences
- Say names of objects
- Imitate parents
- Refer to self by name and use 'me' and 'mine'
- Ask for things ('I want drink')
- Point to eyes, ears, or nose when you ask

## By 3 years of age is the child able to:
*Motor skills*
- Feed self (with some spilling)
- Wash and dry hands by self
- Dress self with help
- Use the toilet with some help
- Walk in a straight line
- Jump with both feet off the ground

*Sensory and thinking skills*
- Recognise sounds in the environment
- Know what is food and what is not food
- Know some numbers (but not always in the right order)
- Know where things usually belong
- Avoid some dangers, such as a hot stove or a moving car
- Follow simple requests

*Language and social skills*
- Use three- to five-word sentences
- Ask short questions

- Name at least ten familiar objects
- Ask to use the toilet almost every time
- Play spontaneously with two or three children in a group
- Assign roles in pretend social play ('You be mummy'; 'I be daddy')
- Know first and last name
- Understand 'I', 'You', 'He' and 'She'

## By 4 years of age, is the child able to:

*Motor skills*
- Hold a pencil
- Draw a circle
- Draw a face
- Pour from a small jug
- Use the toilet alone

*Sensory and thinking skills*
- Understand words such as 'big', 'little', 'tall' and 'short'
- Count up to five objects
- Follow three instructions given at one time (e.g. 'Come inside, wash your hands, and come and eat.')

*Language and social skills*
- Have a large vocabulary
- Want explanations of 'why' and 'how'
- Relate a recent simple experience
- Pretend to play with imaginary objects
- Sometimes cooperate with other children
- Enjoy tag, hide-and-seek and other games with simple rules

## By 5 years of age, is the child able to:

*Gross motor skills*
- Stand on one foot for 10 seconds or longer
- Hop, somersault
- Swing, climb

*Hand and finger skills*
- Copy triangle and other patterns
- Draw person with body
- Dress and undress without assistance
- Usually care for own toilet needs

*Language skills*
- Recall part of a story
- Speak sentences of more than five words
- Use future tense

*Cognitive skills*
- Count ten or more objects
- Correctly name at least four colours
- Know about things used every day in the home (e.g. cooking utensils, food)

*Social and emotional skills*
- Want to please friends
- Want to be like his friends
- Able to distinguish fantasy from reality

## 4.2 Language delay

**Case 4.1**

Five-year-old Ajit has been sent to the clinic by the teacher at the village school where he has just started because he seems to have very few words and the teacher thinks he may have an intellectual disability. Ajit comes with his mother, a small, poorly dressed lady who also brings along two younger children, including a baby who looks unwashed. It turns out she also has three older children at school that day. Ajit's mother does not think there is a problem. Ajit did not speak a single word until he was 3 years old, but he now speaks as well as her other children did at this age. Ajit's father, she says, is a very quiet man who hardly speaks at all, but he is in regular work as a farm labourer. Ajit is a friendly boy who smiles at the health professional and seems very close to his mother. The health professional asks him to draw a man. His drawing has legs, arms and a face with eyes, nose, ears and mouth – quite good for a boy of his age. Yet clearly his language is indeed very limited. When asked to tell the health professional about a picture of a school classroom, he just says 'school' and 'lady' pointing to the teacher. What should the health professional do?

### 4.2.1 Information about language delay

- Language delay should be judged against the range of normal development of the understanding and expression of language.
- Language understanding is nearly always in advance of expression.
- Around 1 year, a child can understand 'No' and 'Pick up' if he has dropped something. He can probably say 'Mama' and 'Bye'.
- Around 2 years he can probably understand 'Go and bring a plate' and 'Show me your nose'. He can probably say 'More' and 'All gone' at the end of his meal. He can ask for things with a single word, for example 'Drink' or 'Biccy' (or a similar word for biscuit).

Table 4.1 lists some reasons why children are not speaking at all by 3 years.

If other causes are ruled out, then the problem is specific language delay. The problem is shown by very limited understanding and vocabulary. This occurs more commonly in children from large, disadvantaged families. Their parents have not been able to give them the same level of care as parents from more advantaged backgrounds. They have been deprived of attention and stimulation. If they are also behind with tasks that do not require language, such as the ability to do things with their hands or draw, then they probably have an intellectual disability. This requires a different approach (see Chapter 5).

Delay in spoken language is very likely to be followed by problems in learning to read (see Section 4.4). Language delay is often accompanied by emotional and/or behaviour problems.

### 4.2.2 Finding out more about children with language delay

- First assess whether the child's language is delayed beyond the normal range. Assess separately what the child can understand and what the child can say.
- If language development is delayed, consider the various possible causes (Table 4.1).

Table 4.1 Differential diagnosis of language delay

| | Intellectual disability | Specific language delay | Deafness | Autism | Selective mutism |
|---|---|---|---|---|---|
| Non-verbal ability | Poor | Average or above average | Average or above average | Average or below average | Average |
| Response to sounds | Normal for developmental level | Normal | Absent or poor | Variable | Normal |
| Use of gesture | Present | Present | Markedly present | Absent or impaired | Present |
| Neologisms (invented words) and echolalia (automatic repeating of words) | Absent or only present briefly | Absent or only present briefly | Absent | Present | Absent |
| Variability in language use | Absent | Absent | Absent | Present | Present |
| Speech intonation | Normal or immature | Often immature | Abnormal | Abnormal | Normal |

Turk *et al* (2007).

- If the child is behind in other areas of development, then the child may have intellectual disability.
- The child's hearing should be carefully tested to rule out deafness (see Section 12.3) as well as other ear problems such as infection (otitis media) or middle ear effusion (glue ear).
- If the child is showing little interest in forming relationships with others and has odd movements, such as hand-flapping, then the child probably has ASD (see Section 4.6).
- If the child is not speaking at school but is speaking at home, then the child has selective mutism (see p. 63).
- If the above are all ruled out, then the language delay is specific and can be managed as below.

Now using the information you have obtained from the child with a language problem and the family member(s) you have seen, try to understand what has happened and decide what is the best course of action.

## 4.2.3 *Helping children with language delay*

Once the problem of language delay has been identified, it is important to try to improve language development as soon as possible. Language delay is a serious barrier to learning in school generally. Unfortunately there is no medical treatment for this problem and in most cases it is unlikely that the health professional will be able to refer to a speech and language therapist, but, of course, if one is available, then a referral should be made.

All the same, there is a great deal that can be done by parents and teachers to promote language development (see Section 15.4). Promoting language should start shortly after birth when shared communication begins while feeding is taking place. The mother can talk to the baby, notice when he has had enough and pause; and use his signals to decide when to go on. A little later when the baby starts to babble, the mother can enter into little pretend conversations, responding to him when he makes sounds and then waiting for him to continue his babbling. Gradually, as his first words appear, the parent needs to respond, correct if he does not get the word quite right, but above all, listen to his attempts to communicate. A little later, parents can use the following tips to encourage language:

- talk to him about what he is doing
- ask him to tell them what he is doing
- ask him what things, such as a cup or a spoon, are used for
- help him to learn what words such as 'Up' and 'Down', 'Over' and 'Under', 'Above' and 'Below' mean
- help him to make comparisons, such as 'Where is the biggest tree?'

Playing games with children and talking at the same time is a good way to encourage language development. Going shopping provides many opportunities for this too, as does watching television by making it an active experience by encouraging the child to talk about what he sees. Telling stories to the child is more likely to help language development if he is engaged in adding to the story or (if it is a familiar story) recounting what is going to happen next.

Brothers and sisters may seem to take up parents' time so that the parents have less time to spend with the child with a problem. But brothers and sisters can be encouraged to listen to and talk with the child who is behind in language so that they actually become helpful. If they are available, grandparents and other relatives can also play their part.

If there are associated behaviour or emotional problems, then these will need attention (see Chapters 7 and 8).

Now, given this information, what can the health professional do to help Ajit, whose story began this section?

## 4.3 Stammering

### 4.3.1 Information about stammering

Stammering means the same as stuttering. The child's speech lacks fluency because of hesitations, repetitions of certain sounds (especially some consonants such as p, t and b) and prolongations of sounds. There may be occasional blocking of (inability to articulate) whole words. Stammering runs in families, with some children more genetically vulnerable than others. There is no particular form of child-rearing that produces stammering, so it is not true to say that parents cause this condition. Apart from the genetic influence, the cause is unknown. It used to be thought that left-handed children were more prone to stammer, especially if an unwise attempt was made to change their handedness. This is no longer thought to be the case.

Stammering usually begins at 3–5 years and is relatively common at this age. Stammering at this early age usually stops completely without treatment, although some speech therapists believe that it is more likely to improve if the child is given treatment. When the stammer does not stop by 5 or 6 years, it may affect the child's life in school very profoundly. The child may be teased by other children and, occasionally, even by teachers.

There is no particular link with behaviour or emotional disorders, but stress at school may result in the child playing truant.

If specialist treatment by a speech and language therapist is available, this may produce some improvement but it will not result in a cure. There is no effective medication, although drugs used to relieve anxiety may be used when a child or adolescent is faced with a situation in which it is felt it is important for him to speak fluently.

**Case 4.2**

Rishi was a 6-year-old boy brought to the clinic by his father because of his stammer. This had been present from the age of 3 years. The stammer affected him in school because he was teased about it. His father said that he had tried shouting at him and hitting him, but this only seemed to make the stammer worse and so he had stopped doing this. Rishi's stammer was quite severe and it took him longer than normal to read a passage in a book. Rishi was a quiet, rather unhappy boy, who did not like to hear his father talk about his stammer. What should the health professional do?

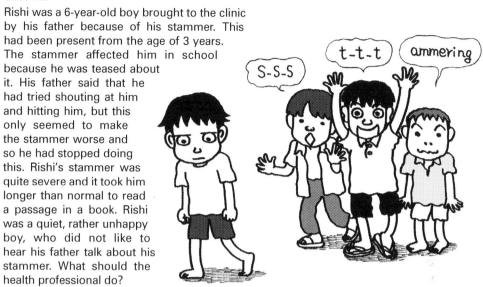

## 4.3.2 Finding out more about children who stammer

- Find out when the stammer began and what, if anything, seemed to have triggered it.
- Find out the situations in which the stammer is better and when it is at its worst. Talking to the child about the stammer may make it worse, but it may, all the same, be necessary to ask the child directly about his problem. He may reveal, for example, that if he stops thinking about it, the stammer is much reduced.
- Ask whether anyone else in the family has stammered.
- Ask how the parents behave when the child stammers. Do they ignore it or try to get him to stop it?
- Is the child teased at home or at school because of his stammer?
- How much does the stammer affect the child's life?
- Are there any behaviour and emotional problems present?

Now using the information you have obtained from the child who has the stammer and the family member(s) you have seen, try to understand what has happened and decide what is the best course of action.

## 4.3.3 Helping children who stammer

- Parents should be encouraged:
  - not to blame themselves – they did not cause the stammer
  - to reassure the child that the stammer is not the child's fault – you know he is doing his best
  - to listen very attentively to what the child says; if the child thinks you are not really listening, the stammer may get worse
  - to help others to behave appropriately to the child with a stammer

- not to make the child speak unnecessarily but always let the child speak if it is clear he wants to say something
- to report any teasing or bullying complaints to his teachers
- to treat their child with the same level of affection and the same degree of discipline as they would a child without a stammer.

- Teachers should be encouraged:
  - to discuss with the child how he would like to be treated. Would he prefer, for example, not to be asked to read aloud or to be allowed to read less than the others? This question may need to be asked more than once in case the child has changed his mind. Reading aloud at home in front of a mirror or to familiar people may help the child to build confidence;
  - to strongly discourage any teasing or bullying, explaining to other children how painful this is to children with a stammer;
  - to encourage the child with a stammer to report any teasing or bullying;
  - to make sure the child is stretched, but not over-stretched, academically.

- Children should be encouraged:
  - to take their time if they have something to say
  - to tell their parents if they would like them to react differently to their stammer
  - to tell their teachers or ask their parents to tell their teachers if they would like different reactions to their stammer
  - to report any teasing or bullying at school to their parents
  - to speak slowly and to practice deep breathing – taking a deep breath is particularly helpful at the start of a sentence or when the child gets stuck on a word
  - practice reading aloud slowly.

If there is any specialist help available from speech and language therapists, then the child should be referred when the stammer has been present for 6 months or more. Earlier referrals result in specialist time being given to children who would have got better anyway. Later referrals may make treatment less effective as the stammer has become established.

Now make a list of the ways in which the health professional might be able to help Rishi.

## 4.4 Reading difficulties

### 4.4.1 Information about reading

Being able to read is essential for learning. Most children begin to learn to read between 5 and 7 years of age, but some do not start until 8 or 9 years. Before they begin to read, they have already learned skills essential for reading:

- understanding and expression of language
- ability to tell the difference between shapes.

Learning to read requires other skills:

- linking different shapes to different sounds
- being able to blend individual sounds into words.

Most children begin to read by making out the sounds of letters. Then they go on to learn how to use the meaning of what they are reading so that they can make out whole words. They may also use the pictures in books to help them 'guess' what the next words are likely to be. Children use a variety of strategies to help them to read successfully. All children need encouragement.

**Case 4.3**
David is a 10-year-old boy whose mother brings him to the clinic because he is always getting stomach aches before going to school. His mother knows what the problem really is – he hates going to school because he cannot read like the other boys. David likes drawing which he is pretty good at and enjoys making things out of discarded plastic pots, but he just cannot read. His mother thinks he sits at the back of the class at school so that he will not get asked any questions or, worse still, asked to read aloud in front of the class. David's two older sisters are reading well, but his father also had difficulty in learning to read and cannot read fluently even now. There is no psychologist available in the locality. What should the health professional do?

## 4.4.2 Information about reading difficulties

There are two main groups of children who have difficulty reading:

1  children who have intellectual disability who have difficulties learning everything or most things (see Chapter 5)
2  children of normal intelligence who only have difficulties in learning to read (dyslexia).

There are various reasons why children of normal intelligence find it difficult to read.

- Genetic influences.
- Problems in the child, including language delay, hearing difficulties, difficulties in telling the differences between shapes, difficulties in linking shapes to sounds, difficulties in blending sounds, difficulties in differentiating between letters and numbers that look similar (e.g. 'b' and 'd'; '6' and '9'). The latter is called 'mirror' reading or writing as children often mistake one for the other.
- Problems in the family, including lack of encouragement to read, little time spent with the child as the parents are too busy, and little conversation between the parents and the child. These problems often arise from poverty, overcrowding and poor educational level of the parents, especially the mother.
- Poor teaching at school caused by too many children in the class or by unskilled teachers.

In children of normal intelligence who have difficulty reading, many more boys than girls are affected and most children go on to have problems in spelling later on. Rates of difficulties in attention and concentration and other behaviour problems are high, as is the rate of language delay and clumsiness (motor coordination disorder).

### 4.4.3 Finding out more about children with reading difficulties

The health professional should check the child's hearing and vision (see Sections 12.3 and 12.4). Test also for clumsiness (see Section 4.5). Assuming that there are no medically remediable problems, if there is a psychologist or specialist teacher available it will be necessary to make an appropriate referral. In the absence of a psychologist, the health professional should:

- assess the child's ability to read – this can be done with some degree of accuracy if the health professional has three or four books of increasing level of difficulty, ranging from very simple baby books to books for adults, and has a clear idea of the level children should have reached at different ages;
- assess the child's level of understanding and expression of language (see Section 4.1.1);
- assess the child's general level of ability (see Section 4.1.1);
- decide whether the child's level of reading ability is about what one would expect from their level of general intelligence or whether it is well below this.

Now using the information you have obtained from the child with a reading problem and the family member(s) you have seen, try to understand what has happened and decide what is the best course of action.

### 4.4.4 Helping children of normal ability with reading difficulties

If the child is of normal general ability but is behind in reading, the health professional should discuss the problem with the parents and the child. Explain that the child does not have a medical but an educational problem. Encourage them to read to the child, tell the child stories, and get the child to talk about pictures in books. Do not punish for failure, but reward the child for small progress. After obtaining permission from the parents, discuss the problem with the child's teachers. Find out whether the teachers are aware of the problem, and whether they can give the child some extra help, and so avoid humiliating the child by asking him to read in front of the class.

Give the child individual support for reading and allow them to build up confidence on simpler words and sentences which are below their level of ability and age.

Now, given this information, what can the health professional do to help David?

## 4.5 Clumsiness

**Case 4.4**

Abhilash is a 9-year-old boy brought by his father to the clinic because he complains of nausea and he cries every morning saying he does not want to go to school. His father thinks that the problem is to do with Abhilash's writing. Whenever the teacher asks the class to write something down, he takes one look at Abhilash's work and laughs at him. Often, the teacher, who is very keen on good, neat handwriting, asks 'How am I supposed to read this scribble?'. Now Abhilash, who has always seemed a bright boy, does not want to go to school and says he feels like vomiting nearly every weekday morning. His parents think this is a fairly obvious excuse. The health professional found out that Abhilash walked and talked at the usual times. His speech was a little slow to develop and he had some difficulty in making himself understood. His attention span is a little short but he can concentrate in the classroom. He has always been a clumsy child. He did not manage to handle a cup properly until he was 4 years old. He is still clumsy using a spoon and food spills off his plate when he eats. He is not very good at ball games. He can run quite fast but he looks awkward when he is running. He still cannot catch a ball. When he tries to kick a ball he often falls over and the other boys laugh at him. He is always the last to be chosen when the children pick teams.

## 4.5.1 Information about clumsiness

Other terms for clumsiness include dyspraxia and developmental coordination disorder. More boys than girls are found to be clumsy but this may be because boys are expected to be more agile and sporty.

Clumsiness usually shows itself in the first 3 or 4 years of life. Children may be slow to walk, and then have difficulty in holding a cup or spoon. They may bump into things and fall over a lot. They are slow to dress themselves and have particular difficulty doing up buttons or shoelaces. Once they start school they will have problems with handwriting and this may cause them trouble in most school subjects. Often it is only by school age that it becomes obvious that a child's slightly clumsy movements are not just a development phase but are beginning to be a significant problem.

Clumsiness is mainly caused by genetic influences. Very occasionally the problem may be caused by a neuromuscular disorder or by medication the child is taking. Children born very prematurely are more at risk, but most children who are clumsy have been born following a normal delivery.

The type of clumsiness may not be easy to detect. Some children seem to have a poor sense of the position of their limbs (known as proprioception). This is something most children have automatically. Others have difficulties in recognising when the patterns they are making or drawing are the same or different (perceptual or spatial difficulties). Obviously this will cause problems in handwriting. A child may not be able to tell the difference between a 'b' and a 'd' or between a 'p' and a 'q' and so have a problem learning to read.

There is a link with overactivity and attention problems (see Section 8.2). Children who have severe or moderate learning difficulties or ASD are also often clumsy. However, most children who are clumsy are of normal intelligence.

Children who are clumsy often have a poor opinion of themselves. Boys especially may become depressed because they are not nearly as good as other children at sport. They may develop oppositional behaviour as they resent being told off particularly when they are trying hard.

Children who are clumsy in the first few years of life are likely to remain so during childhood and adolescence, but they can be helped in a number of ways.

## 4.5.2 Finding out more about children who are clumsy

- Obtain an account of the problems the child is having, especially in writing and in sporting activities. If the child is old enough, make sure the child is involved in giving the story.
- Find out about any early problems in coordination, for example in holding a cup and eating with a spoon.
- Ask whether the child has any problems in attention or concentration in school.
- Ask how the child is affected by his clumsiness – does it make him miserable or anxious?
- Examine the child for muscle weakness or any other obvious neurological disorder.
- Observe the child walking along a straight line and hopping. Get them to touch their fingers in turn against the thumb of the same hand. Watch the child's handwriting yourself. Get the child to throw and catch a ball. Judge the child's performance in these tasks against how other children you know or have seen can perform.

- If possible, discuss the child's clumsiness with the school and find out how they think the child is affected.
- Decide with the parent(s) and child whether the child really is unusually clumsy.
- Note, a child's clumsiness if often very variable: a child might appear quite able one day, but another day, especially if tired, might have a lot more difficulty. Many children who are clumsy can perform quite well on some tasks such as handwriting if they try hard for short periods of time (e.g. when being examined) but cannot keep up the effort.

Now, given the information you have obtained from observing the child and talking to the family member(s), try to understand why the child is so clumsy. Then go on to work out a plan to help.

## 4.5.3 Helping children who are clumsy

Assuming the child is unusually clumsy but, as is nearly always the case, there is no neurological problem present, explain to the parent(s) and child what the problem is. Explain (if this is indeed the case) that you do not really know why the child is unusually clumsy but that some children are born this way. Always add that this does not mean there is nothing that can be done to help – indeed, although there is no cure, there is a lot that can be done. If the child has an associated problem with attention or concentration refer to Section 8.2 for what to do.

Explain to the child's school about the nature of the child's clumsiness and encourage the teachers to take a sympathetic attitude to the problem. It is not the child's fault. The parents are probably already sympathetic but may need to be talked to along similar lines.

There are three approaches to helping the child with the difficulties he is experiencing as a result of clumsiness. They should all be used. First, the child needs more practice than others in the tasks he finds difficult. It is really important to give the child more opportunities to practice handwriting than is the case with other children. Parents can practice throwing, catching and kicking a ball. This should be seen as fun, not as a task to be completed. Often running, jumping, swinging and catching a big ball are both fun and the best way of helping develop coordination for more precise tasks such as handwriting.

Second, the child needs to be helped to find alternative activities to those which he finds a problem, so sports that do not require as much coordination as others, such as running rather than football, are to be preferred. As computers gradually become universally available, even to children in LAMI countries, handwriting will become less important. Children with handwriting problems need to be given more time to complete tasks.

Third, boost the child's confidence by making sure he gets lots of praise just for trying hard as well as for making small improvements in the things he is not good at. Encourage the child to talk about his feelings if he is left out of team games and find other things for him to do instead.

It is very unlikely that there will be any specialist therapists, such as occupational therapists, available to advise, but if there are then a referral should be made. A great deal of help can, however, be given by parents and teachers.

Now make a list of the ways in which the health professional might be able to help Abhilash.

# 4.6 Autism spectrum disorder

**Case 4.5**

Mustafa is a 4-year-old boy whose mother is very worried because he has no speech. He has never said a word. He does not seem to understand speech either. He does not respond when he is called by his name. He does seem to respond to sounds he has not heard before and is upset by loud noises. He is unusual in other ways too. He does not look at his mother in the face when she talks to him. He seems to want to look away. Unlike her second child who is now 2 years old, he does not like to be picked up and cuddled, and struggles to be put down. In fact he has never seemed to miss his mother when she is not there. Even when he hurts himself he does not look to his mother to comfort him. He also has a strange way of flapping his hands up and down when he is excited. Yet Mustafa started to walk by himself quite normally when he was 1 year old and he is able to draw a man, using a pencil, better than most 4-year-olds.

**Case 4.6**

Josef is a 10-year-old boy whose teachers have told his mother to take him to the health professional because they think he is very odd. His mother is not too worried about him, although she recognises that he is an unusual boy. He looks away when looked in the eye. He does not have any friends and does not seem to mind this. He is very close to his mother. His speech is also unusual because although he uses language correctly, he speaks in a rather mechanical way, almost as if he were a machine or a robot. His schoolwork is good, especially his number work. Indeed, he is unusually good with his numbers and can multiply numbers together much better than most children of his age.

Both of these boys have language development and relationship problems. They both have autism spectrum disorder (ASD), with Mustafa at the severe end of the spectrum and Josef at the milder end. Josef's condition is sometimes called Asperger syndrome, where there is no speech delay and the language is well developed but its use is odd and mechanical.

## 4.6.1 Information about ASD

Children with ASD have problems with their development which is very uneven. Usually this abnormality of development is present from birth, but occasionally development is normal for the first 18 months or 2 years, after which, often for no obvious reason, their development becomes seriously abnormal, with the loss of some of the skills they had achieved.

### Social development

Relationships with other people are both delayed and abnormal. If severely affected, children with ASD are very slow to become attached to their mother and other family members. They do not seem to show any anxiety when they are separated from their mother. Such separation anxiety is a feature of normal development, especially between the ages of 6 and 18 months (see Chapter 15). Gradually, such children do become attached to members of their family and may become quite clingy by the age of 5 or 6 years. Less severely affected children do show some affection and sociability with close family members but do not develop friendships with other children. They seem to like being solitary. Others appear to try to play with other children but hit them or say upsetting things and then find it difficult to understand why the other children are upset or do not want to play with them.

### Language development

For some severely affected children, spoken language never develops at all. Others do develop speech but in an unusual way, for example they may echo or repeat back words that are spoken to them (echolalia) and make up words they have never heard (neologisms). They might, for example, call a chair a 'sit-down'. More mildly affected children often have normal language except for their intonation – the way they pronounce their words is often monotonous and mechanical sounding or may have special accents.

### Odd interests

More severely affected children easily become obsessed with apparently meaningless rituals such as spinning things around. More able children may have well-developed but unusual interests, for example in maps or timetables. They often have difficulty understanding that other people do not share their interests.

### Odd movements

Odd movements (the most common is flapping of the hands) are called mannerisms or stereotypies and are likely to be most obvious when the child is excited or upset. Mildly affected children may not show these at all.

### Sensitivity to noise

If there is a loud noise, more severely affected children may put their hands up to their ears as if they are in pain.

### Frequency

Boys are affected four or five times more than girls. The severe form of ASD is rather rare, occurring in about 1 in 3000 children. The milder form is much more common, occurring in as many as 1 per 100–200 children.

### Causes

Abnormal genes are by far the most important cause of ASD. Children with ASD sometimes have a parent who is rather solitary. Most brothers and sisters develop normally, but they do have language and other learning problems somewhat more often than siblings of children without ASD. It has not so far been possible to identify the exact genetic abnormality, although a number of genes have been implicated. Occasionally, children with ASD have a rare genetic disorder such as tuberose sclerosis that affects their brain and causes this type of developmental problem.

### Associated problems

Many children with ASD are slow in other aspects of their development such as using a pencil or gaining bladder and bowel control. In contrast, a small minority are unusually gifted in, for example, drawing, music or computers. Children with ASD have a slight but definite increase in the risk of developing epilepsy.

### Outcome

Mildly affected children will improve and be able to lead normal lives, although it is likely they will always have difficulty getting on with other people. More severely affected children will also improve but at a much slower rate. In adulthood they will probably only be able to live partly independent lives and will continue to need special care.

Now, given the information you have obtained, try to understand how ASD has arisen in this particular child. Then go on to work out a plan to help.

## 4.6.2 Helping children with ASD

### Need for special upbringing

Children with ASD are different from those with general learning difficulties or intellectual disability. They show average or even occasionally above average ability in some skills, especially drawing, music or computer skills, so they should not be treated in the same way.

### Explanation to parents

Parents, especially mothers, are often particularly confused and upset by the rejecting way these children behave towards them. They need reassurance and to be told that their child's problems are not their fault. They will benefit from continuing support from other family members, friends and health professionals as the child gets older.

### Help but no cure

Medication has no part to play except for associated problems such as epilepsy or hyperactivity (see Sections 8.2 and 12.6). Parents can be helped to cope with their child better, to reduce some of their behaviour problems and to promote their development. If parents name things when they use them – 'drink', 'dinner', 'bed', 'book' – their children may gradually learn what these words mean. Parents should try to communicate in any way possible, including the use of signs. Mildly affected children will be able to attend school, but more severely affected children are likely to have to be kept at home. Parents will need all the help they can get from other family members and friends if they are to continue looking after the child. In most areas there will be no special schools for children with these problems, but if there are, such children should attend.

### Reducing difficult behaviour

Parents should be encouraged to ignore difficult behaviour but to reward all desirable behaviours with words of praise. Hugs and cuddles may not be liked by the child. Observe the child, learn what kind of activities/words makes him happy. Mildly affected children can be helped to get on better with other children if it is realised they need a great deal of help to make friends.

## 4.6.3 Identifying and treating signs and symptoms

Early identification of signs and symptoms (Box 4.1) in the second and third year of life and intensive intervention are important in improving outcome (Bryanne & Eapen, 2012). The 'wait and see' method often recommended to concerned parents could lead to missed opportunities. Instead, pre-school children can be helped through programmes (at home, at school or at special centres) directed at providing intense stimulation with opportunities for play. The main goals include:

1  bringing the child into social relationships rather than allowing the child to drift away from the social circle of the home environment
2  following the child's lead when interacting with the child, and
3  engaging the child in play activities that involve interacting and communicating with the child using the following strategies:
    i    responding sensitively to even the slightest emotional response from the child
    ii   balancing your actions according to the interest shown by the child
    iii  imitating and matching the emotional and social responses of the child
    iv  sharing and turn taking
    v   engaging in activities that promote joint attention where the child attends to an object or event (e.g. 'Hey look…') with another adult (parent, teacher or therapist) in joint activities.

Box 4.1 Early signs and symptoms suggestive of autism

- Does not respond to his name being called or recognise familiar sounds (familiar voice, door-bell, etc.)
- Does not point to or show things as a way of sharing the experience
- Does not use gesture to communicate (e.g. waving bye-bye)
- Does not interact with others during play (e.g. showing or looking up for a reaction) or engage in social games (e.g. peek-a-boo or hide-and-seek)
- Does not engage in pretend play (e.g. feeding doll; racing car) or engage in group games, imitate others, or use toys in creative ways
- Does not let you know what he wants or does not want
- Does not imitate actions (including facial expression) or speech or songs
- Unusual (lining up or spinning objects, moving fingers in front of the eyes) and repetitive behaviours (e.g. hand flapping, rocking, tip-toe walking)
- Does not like to be touched, held or cuddled
- Does not attend jointly with you to share an experience (e.g. does not respond to 'Hey, look….' or bring toys to 'show' you)
- Does not show interest or is unaware of what's going on around
- Does not know how to connect with others, or make friends
- Does not understand other people's feelings, intentions, etc.
- Restricted interests, insistence on doing things the same way and does not like change to routines

Speech stimulation (see Section 4.2 on language delay), social skills training and educational programmes ensure optimum development and well-being. Behavioural therapy techniques can help children acquire self-help and social skills and improve communication. Although healthy children learn mostly by observing and through minimal adult guidance the daily living skills such as feeding, dressing and toilet training, as well as social skills such as playing and interacting with others, children with ASD need teaching and training using specific techniques. Similar to those used in intellectual disability, these techniques include:

- rewarding by praising the child and giving rewards when the child shows desirable behaviour or makes an attempt to learn appropriate and new behaviours
- modelling and encouraging the child to do the activity by showing the child how this is done
- teaching the simplified version of a complex activity first and then gradually increasing the complexity at a pace comfortable to the child
- teaching an activity such as feeding skills by breaking it up into several small steps (see Section 5.3 on helping children with intellectual disability) – this can be done by starting with the first step and going forwards or teaching the last step first and then going backwards
- for children who are not able to learn by modelling, the child can be taught the activity by holding their hands and doing it with them until they are able to do it by themselves.

Now work out ways in which a health professional could help Mustafa and Josef.

# CHAPTER 5

# Intellectual disability

**Case 5.1**

Ranjit was brought by his father to the clinic because Ranjit was very slow to learn. At 5 years most of his skills were more like those of a boy half his age. He had only just learned to feed himself with a spoon. He still soiled and wet himself day and night. His language was more like that of a 2-year-old. He could say single words but had no sentences. He had been able to walk by 18 months and, although he was a bit floppy, his leg and arm movements were more or less up to his age level. No one else in the family had been slow to learn. His father was a junior clerk in the civil service. Ranjit's behaviour was generally good. He was an obedient, rather passive boy. What should the health professional do?

## 5.1 Information about intellectual disability[1]

In Chapter 4 we described children whose development was slow in just one or two areas. In this chapter we describe children whose development is slow or very slow in all or nearly all areas.

As children grow older, they develop a range of abilities, skills and capacities, and become more adapted to their environments. The main skills acquired are to do with movement, language and social relationships. Some are slower to acquire these skills than others and some children never acquire skills at an adult level.

Children whose abilities are at or below the level of children half their age have severe intellectual disability. Children who are more intelligent than this but are only at or below the level of children about three-quarters of their age have mild intellectual disability. For example, a 12-year-old child who is functioning at or below the level of a 6-year-old has severe intellectual disability. A 12-year-old child who is at a level between 6 and 9 years old has mild intellectual disability. A child of 12 years who is at a 9- to 11-year level may be a little slow but is within the normal range. Severe and, to a lesser degree, mild intellectual disability affect the way children function in a variety of ways:

- ability to walk and use hands
- self-care, such as feeding, washing, using the toilet independently
- talking and understanding language
- social functioning, such as playing with other children.

The more severe the intellectual disability, the more difficult it will be for the child to carry out these various functions.

---

1. The terms mental retardation/learning difficulties/intellectual disability are used interchangeably in different regions of the world.

## 5.1.1 Causes

In children with severe and mild intellectual disability the brain is not working as well as it should. There are various reasons why the brain does not develop and work properly.

Most children with severe intellectual disability have abnormal genes or chromosomes affecting the brain, a very large number of which have been identified. Most common is an abnormality on chromosome 21 causing Down syndrome, which is responsible for causing about a third of severe intellectual disability in high-income countries, although less than this in LAMI countries, where other causes (listed below) are more prevalent. Women over the age of 35 years are at higher risk of giving birth to babies with Down syndrome. Some children with Down syndrome fall into the mild intellectual disability category. There are many other genetic causes, most of which are uncommon or rare.

Brain damage before, during or after birth may also be responsible. While the baby is in the womb, damage to the brain can occur if the mother is poorly nourished, drinks an excessive amount of alcohol, has a diet deficient in iodine or, because of damage to the placenta, the blood supply to the fetus is inadequate. The brain may be damaged at birth during the passage of the baby through the birth canal, or if immediately after birth the baby's breathing is delayed for some reason, or by an illness after birth. If the baby is very premature, there may be a bleed (haemorrhage) into the brain. Severe jaundice or meningitis may also damage the brain. If the child is neglected after birth, understimulated, undernourished or abused in other ways, the brain will not develop properly. This is a common cause of mild intellectual disability. Note that often there is more than one cause.

In most cases there is an identifiable cause for severe intellectual disability, although this is less often the case for mild intellectual disability. However, identifying a cause may require expensive equipment. Most of the causes identified by the use of such equipment are not treatable, so lack of such equipment does not mean that children with intellectual disability are deprived of a cure.

Children with severe intellectual disability and, to a lesser extent, mild intellectual disability have an increased likelihood of developing an emotional or behaviour problem. Difficulties with attention and concentration are especially common, but these children are also more likely to have anxiety and depressive states and aggressive behaviour. There is a small number of behaviour problems such as self-injury which virtually only occur in children with severe intellectual disability. Children with severe intellectual disability and, to a lesser extent, mild intellectual disability are at greater risk of epilepsy (see Section 12.6). They are also at greater risk of other physical problems such as hearing and visual impairment.

## 5.1.2 Impact of severe intellectual disability on the child and family

- Children with severe intellectual disability will remain dependent on their parents for much longer than 'normal' children, quite possibly for the whole of their lives.
- There will be an economic impact on the family. The child will not be able to contribute to the family income. One parent may have to stay at home and, in the absence of a member of the extended family who can look after the child, not be able to go out to work.
- In many localities, children with severe intellectual disability will not be allowed to go to school, thus restricting the child's ability to learn.
- Parents may experience guilt and shame at the presence of a child with severe intellectual disability who will or may look different from other children. Sometimes parents may 'hide' such children from society.

- The child may be stigmatised in the neighbourhood, teased and bullied. If the child does go to school, he may be similarly picked on and called names.
- The life expectancy of children with severe intellectual disability is significantly reduced.

### 5.1.3 *Impact of mild intellectual disability on the child and family*

- The child will gradually be able to achieve independence, although more slowly than other children.
- In most areas the child will be able to go to school and, after leaving school, will be able to find employment in an unskilled job.
- This means that the impact on the family will be much less than with children with severe intellectual disability.
- Children with mild intellectual disability will probably be able to hold down an unskilled job, marry and have children. They will probably have normal or near normal life expectancy.

## 5.2 Finding out more about children with intellectual disability

You should suspect the presence of intellectual disability when a child:

- is slow to pass most or all of the milestones at the usual ages (see Section 4.1)
- is having difficulty in schoolwork
- is not as independent or as capable of self-help as other children.

If you suspect intellectual disability you should try and work out at what age level the child is functioning in different areas, such as movement, language and social relationships. Then find out at what ages the child passed the various milestones.

Remember that the child may not be functioning at an age-appropriate level because his parents are overprotective and do not allow him to do various things. Try to establish at what age level the child is functioning in movement (including coordination of hands and fingers), language and social relationships (see Section 4.1), as well as in self-care. If the child is at school, ask the teacher what level he thinks the child is at, or get a school report. In some situations, children do not achieve as well as parents think they should. Parents may be right to worry about this, but sometimes their children are not as intelligent as they think they are. Information from both the parents and the teacher about the child's functioning in different settings and for different tasks would be helpful in determining what is causing the child to underachieve.

Assuming the child is showing severe or mild intellectual disability, try to establish a cause, first by taking a history.

- Ask the parents whether anyone else in the family has been slow to learn.
- Ask whether the pregnancy was normal. Was there any bleeding during the pregnancy? Did the mother have an adequate diet? Did she drink alcohol, and if so, how much?
- What was the birth like? How long did it last? Was it necessary to use forceps or to deliver by Caesarean section? Were there any other complications? How much did the baby weigh at birth? Did the baby cry and breathe straight away or was there a delay?
- Has the child had any illnesses after birth? In particular, did the child have any brain infections?
- Is there any history of trauma to the brain? Has the child had any accidents, been dropped, etc?
- Has the child had any fits/seizures?

Then examine the child to see whether this can give a clue to the cause of the intellectual disability. Most children with mild intellectual disability look normal. Some children with severe intellectual disability may have an unusual appearance which can provide clues; for example, children with Down syndrome have slanting eyes, low ears, a short neck, a small mouth so that the tongue looks large and may stick out, and a single crease across the palms of their hands. Examine the child fully for evidence of other health problems. In particular, test the child for deafness and for eyesight problems (see Sections 12.3 and 12.4).

If the child's language and social development are well behind his ability to draw, and he is very sensitive to noise and has unusual habits, such as flapping of the hands, think of the possibility that he has ASD (see pp. 25–28). Of course, he may have intellectual disability as well. If the child is generally at the level of other children of his age but is very behind in language, he may have a specific language delay (see pp. 16–18). Also, if the child is underachieving in school-related skills but on par with other areas of development, it may be a specific reading disability/dyslexia or other learning problems and not intellectual disability. Similarly, if the child is generally at the level of other children but has very poor movement coordination, this may require further physical and neurological assessments.

It is worth looking for bruising of the skin or other signs of maltreatment, as children with severe intellectual disability are at particular risk of being abused.

Note that if there is one available, you should refer to a child health specialist to confirm your view and to carry out investigations, especially biochemical studies, neuroimaging and chromosome analysis that will not be possible in a health clinic. The results will not lead to a cure, but will mean that the parents have a better idea of the cause of their child's problem. This may help to give a better idea of the risk of abnormality if they are planning further children.

Now using the information you have obtained from your observations of the child with intellectual disability and from talking with the family member(s) you have seen, try to understand what has caused the problem, how it is affecting the lives of the child and family members, and decide what is the best course of action.

## 5.3 Helping children with intellectual disability

First, it is important to be sure that the child has an intellectual disability. Then, using the above criteria you should try to decide what level of disability the child has – mild or severe. Below the age of 5 years, although you can be sure of the presence of severe intellectual disability, it may be more difficult to decide whether the child has mild intellectual disability.

If the child has severe intellectual disability, you will first need to break the news to the parents. Remember to ask them first what they think the matter is with the child. They may well have realised their child is very slow to develop. You will need to explain to the parents that their child has an intellectual disability. If the child has severe intellectual disability, it is very likely he will continue to be very slow to develop. The child will do more every year but will remain slow and behind other children of the same age. Explain that there is no cure for intellectual disability but that there is a great deal that parents can do to improve the child's quality of life. The following are useful tips for parents of children with intellectual disability.

- Treat the child according to the child's mental age, not according to the actual age. So if the child is 4 years old but is behaving like a 2-year-old and has only developed to a 2-year level, talk to and play with the child as if he were 2 years old.
- Use praise and rewards for very small progress. Punishment is not likely to be effective.
- Always expect the child to do just a little bit more than he is doing at the present time, in self-help, in language and in achieving control of his bladder and bowel.

- Teach the child how to do things in small steps. For example, if you are teaching the child how to use a spoon to feed, first get the child used to the feel of a spoon, then get the child to scoop food up with a spoon, and finally encourage the child to move the spoon with food on it towards his mouth.
- Try to persuade the teachers to take the child into school. With a child with mild intellectual disability, this will not usually be a problem, but teachers may not like to have a child with severe intellectual disability in the classroom. All the same, it is helpful even for children with severe intellectual disability to attend school. If by chance there is a special school for children with severe intellectual disability, this will be ideal, but this is not likely to be the case in most localities.
- Encourage parents not to neglect their other children. It is easy for parents to give all their attention to the child with intellectual disability. This is not helpful for the other children, who may develop emotional or behaviour problems if they are neglected.
- Brothers and sisters can be encouraged to help so that all the burden does not fall on the parents. Conversely, in some families, the brothers and sisters may feel left out as all the care seems to be given to the child with intellectual disability.
- Encourage parents also not to neglect their own needs. Parents who sacrifice everything for their child with a disability may become angry and frustrated. They should try to find some time for themselves.
- If the child has a behaviour or emotional problem, assess and manage the child as described in other sections of this manual.
- As far as possible, the child should be encouraged to mix with other children. This will be more difficult as the child gets older unless there are other children with intellectual disability in the locality.

As children with severe intellectual disability move into adolescence, they may develop other problems.

- They are at increased risk of psychosis (see p. 107) and epilepsy (see p. 123).
- There may be problems associated with their sexual development. If they start to masturbate in public they should not be punished, but be gently encouraged to do this only in private.
- If they start to make sexual advances to other children or adults it should be made clear to them that this is not acceptable.
- As their formal education is likely to have finished by now, they should be given simple and, if possible, useful tasks to perform to keep them busy, and made to feel they are contributing to the family.

When talking with the parents, always remember to keep the child in the picture and try to talk to the child as well. Remember children with mild and even severe intellectual disability can often understand or communicate their needs more than you think, so listen and talk with the child as much as is possible. Finally, remember that the parents will most likely experience shame and guilt about the fact that they have a child with intellectual disability. They should be given the opportunity to express their feelings.

Now make a list of the ways in which the health professional might be able to help Ranjit.

# CHAPTER 6

# Habit disorders

Habit disorders include:

- feeding problems for which there is no physical cause – the baby may refuse the breast or bottle, fail to suck, cry before or after feeds, have constipation or diarrhoea, vomit or appear to have abdominal pain. Later the young child may fail to thrive for non-organic reasons;
- sleep problems – the child may have difficulty settling at bedtime, may wake frequently during the night, or may wake very early in the morning and disturb the household. As a result of being awake some of the night, the child may be tired during the day. Much less commonly the child may sleep excessively during the day. There may be other problems related to sleep in the early years, such as sleep-walking, nightmares and night terrors;
- bladder and bowel problems, especially bed-wetting and soiling;
- tics and other movement disorders.

## 6.1 Feeding problems

**Case 6.1**
Benjamin is a 2-year-old boy brought by his grandmother to the clinic because he has been refusing to eat his food from the first few weeks of life. The grandmother explains that Benjamin's mother is lying in bed – she has difficulty in getting up in the morning. There is no father in the home. Benjamin is apathetic when he is presented with food and turns his head away. He seems to prefer to watch the television. His development is a little delayed. He is walking well, but is only saying a few single words. When he is weighed and measured, he is below the second centile in both height and weight. The food supply in the area is more than adequate. What should the health professional do?

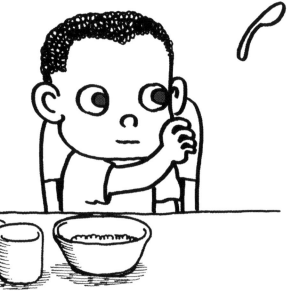

## 6.1.1 Feeding problems in the first 3 months of life

These are likely to be due to:

- exclusive breastfeeding: poor fixation or breast sepsis or maternal illness, especially HIV infection, tuberculosis, depression and chronic infectious disease
- too early introduction of complementary feeding, leading to infection or inadequate calorie intake
- illness in the child such as neonatal tetanus, pertussis and other congenital abnormalities.

Where there is enough food in a locality, there are other reasons for feeding problems in young infants.

- Problems in the baby such as inability to suck as a result of an anatomical abnormality of the mouth, tongue or other part of the swallowing apparatus, or because of brain damage. The baby may be temperamentally very restless or apathetic or may cry persistently after feeds. There may be a physical illness such as a congenital heart condition, cystic fibrosis, anaemia or narrowing of the gullet or narrowing of the outlet from the stomach (pyloric stenosis).
- Problems in the mother, such as an abnormality of the breast or nipple (uncommon), anxiety leading to clumsy handling of the baby, or depressive feelings with apathy and lack of interest in the baby.
- Problems in the feeding technique with, for example, the baby being held too close or too far away from the breast, or, with bottle feeding, too large or too small an opening in the teat.
- Problems in the mother–baby relationship. Successful early feeding needs the establishment of a rhythm between mother and baby, with both satisfying each other's needs. Too frequent or too infrequent feeds, for example, may lead to a breakdown of the feeding relationship.

## 6.1.2 Feeding problems from 3 months to 3 years: failure to thrive

In many LAMI countries, although the food supply is adequate, the distribution of food is such that people in poorer areas are malnourished. Where the food supply is adequate the following feeding problems may occur:

- finicky eating habits (unusual in LAMI countries)
- overeating
- putting things that are not food (e.g. dirt, grass) into the mouth
- vomiting.

These feeding problems are only important if they lead to a failure to thrive. Children who fail to thrive have fallen below the second centile in height, thus are very small for their age. Failure to thrive always arises from inadequate calorie intake, which in turn may be due to an inadequate food supply. Where the food supply is adequate the main reasons for failure to thrive are:

- physical causes in the child, including chronic infection and, much less commonly, heart failure, food allergies or failure to absorb food
- temperamental characteristics of the child such as an unusual degree of restlessness that makes the child difficult to feed
- poor social conditions, with lack of sanitation, overcrowding and financial hardship
- inadequate parenting, perhaps due to depression in the mother leading to apathy, irritability and insensitivity to the needs of the child

- inappropriate feeding practices – the child may be fed too quickly, with too many distractions such as the television on, or with food that is unattractive, too hot or too cold.

## 6.1.3 Finding out more about children with feeding problems

The health professional should weigh and measure the child, plotting height against weight on a growth chart (www.who.int/childgrowth/standards/en/). There should be a record of the child's height and weight from birth so that a check can be made as to whether the child was growing satisfactorily and then showed growth faltering.

- A physical examination should be carried out to help rule out any form of chronic disease.
- A blood test should be carried out to rule out anaemia.
- Urine should be examined for infection.
- Is there sufficient appropriate food available for the child?
- Is there any evidence of infection, especially chronic infection such as tuberculosis or HIV infection or a combination of these?
- Is the mother physically and mentally fit? In particular, does she have any chronic infectious disease or signs of a depressive disorder?
- If there is appropriate food available and there is no evidence of illness in the child or mother, then:
  - find out when the feeding problem began. Has it been present from birth or developed more recently?
  - what does the feeding problem consist of – rejection of food, overeating, playing with food in the mouth, vomiting, pain with eating?
  - what food is the child being given? Is she being given snacks or food between meals?
  - what is going on during mealtimes? Is the television on? Are other children sitting at table, and if so, are they constantly getting up and down from the table?
  - what has the mother already tried to overcome the feeding difficulty?
  - are there any other problems such as sleeping difficulties?
  - does the mother have a physical or mental health problem? In particular, is she depressed, anxious, worn out by pressures and stress?
  - if a friend or relative is available who knows the mother, ask whether they have any observations about the child's feeding.

The single most useful part of assessment of a feeding problem is direct observation of the mother feeding the child, if at all possible in the home, but if not, in the clinic.

Now, given the information you have obtained, try to understand how the feeding problem has arisen in this particular child. Then go on to work out a plan to help.

## 6.1.4 Helping children with feeding problems

Mothers who complain that their children have feeding difficulties but whose children are not failing to thrive may be given practical advice and reassured that their child does not have a serious health problem.

- If the child is failing to thrive, intervention should be based on the findings on assessment. In LAMI countries, it is most likely that there is not sufficient appropriate food available, the child has an infection or the mother is unwell or exhausted as a result of financial or other stresses.

- If the child is failing to thrive despite the availability of appropriate food and absence of evidence for infection, then observation of the feeding situation in the home is likely to reveal the nature of the problem and to suggest what should be done about it. The following interventions may be appropriate depending on the assessment findings:
  - practical advice to the mother on her feeding technique – this should be followed by repeated observation of her feeding to assess the degree to which the advice has been taken and has been effective
  - appropriate counselling for mental health problems such as depression or anxiety in parents.

Now make a list of the ways in which the health professional might be able to help Benjamin and his grandmother.

## 6.2 Obesity

**Case 6.2**

Alok is brought by his mother at the age of 9 years to the clinic with a recurrent cough. He developed this about 3 weeks ago after a bad cold. The health professional examines the chest and finds nothing wrong. In any case, the cough is getting better. However, the health professional does notice that Alok is very fat. She measures his height and weight and finds he is above the 97th centile for weight. His body mass index (BMI) is 35. She asks his mother whether she is worried about his weight. The mother smiles and says that, of course, she knows he is a bit fat but there is nothing she can do about it. He just loves eating. She herself is overweight and has type 2 diabetes. Apparently there is nothing else the matter with Alok. He is doing well at school. He does have friends, but prefers to stay at home to watch television and DVDs. What should the health professional do?

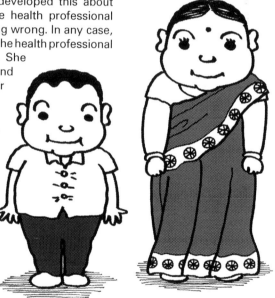

### 6.2.1 Information about obesity

In many middle-income countries, obesity is now a more widespread nutritional problem than malnutrition. Moderate and severe obesity in children are major health problems, predisposing to type 2 diabetes and metabolic syndrome with high BMI, blood pressure and cholesterol levels in adolescence and to the later development of heart disease, respiratory disease, joint problems, varicose veins, poor operative risk and obstructive sleep apnoea.

Hormonal causes of obesity are extremely unusual. If the child is unusually short compared with his parents, this would be worth considering. Sometimes obesity may be part of a chromosomal abnormality (e.g. Prader–Willi syndrome). Most commonly there are just two main causes of obesity and these are usually both present:

1    excessive calorie intake (too much food), and
2    too little exercise.

Some children are genetically predisposed to develop obesity if they eat too much or take too little exercise. They have genes that make it more likely they will turn food into body fat than are other children. Genes have no or little influence on whether a whole population has a high or low prevalence of obesity. Stress during the pregnancy may also make babies more likely to develop obesity later. In addition, bottle-fed babies are more likely to become obese than those who are breast-fed.

Significant reasons for overeating are:

- a family pattern of overeating.
- parents not liking their children to be hungry
- cheapness and ease of access of unhealthy foods
- friends eating unhealthy foods and advertisements on television
- having depression and being apathetic.

Significant reasons for taking too little exercise are:

- watching television and DVDs, playing computer games or 'surfing' on the internet for large amounts of the day
- lack of interest in sport
- a family pattern of inactivity
- social isolation.

Often, children who are depressed may use food for comfort. Obesity may also be a side-effect of some types of medication, especially antipsychotics. Unfortunately, children who are obese are more likely to be unpopular and teased by others.

Most parents of children who are seriously overweight do not ask for help – the obesity is noticed when the child attends for some other reason. The outcome of treatment for obesity is generally poor, especially if children do not see obesity as a problem. Unfortunately, the management programme described below, although it has a small chance of success in highly motivated children, is unlikely to be widely effective unless the parents are highly motivated to change their own lifestyle.

## 6.2.2 Finding out more about children who are obese

Note why the obesity has come to notice. Is this because you have noticed it or because the parents or child want help with it?

Weigh and measure the child. Assess the degree of obesity using growth charts (www.who.int/childgrowth/standards/en/) and/or skin thickness and/or BMI. Body mass index is used to estimate the total amount of body fat and it is calculated by dividing the weight in kilograms (kg) by the height in metres squared ($m^2$). For example, a child who is 35 kg in weight and is 130 cm in height has a BMI of 27 ($35/1.3 = 27$). However, it is to be noted that, unlike in adults, BMI is both age- and gender-specific for children and adolescents as the amount of body fat changes with age and also differs between girls and boys. Therefore the BMI must be compared against age and gender percentile charts (e.g. www.cdc.gov/growthcharts/html_charts/bmiagerev.htm). Similarly, BMI may not correspond to the same degree of obesity in different populations due, in part, to different body proportions. Therefore the health risks associated with BMI score may differ for different populations (http://apps.who.int/bmi/index.jsp?introPage=intro_3.html).

Assuming the child is overweight, assess the attitudes of the child and parents to the problem. Are the parents/child worried at all, slightly or seriously? Remember that the attitudes of the child and parents are a better guide to action than the degree of obesity as you measure it.

Take a rough dietary history and test the child's urine for sugars. Taking an accurate dietary history is not possible without specialist dietary resources, but you can find out what sort of foods the child prefers and whether the child snacks between meals. In addition, make a rough assessment of the amount of exercise the child is taking. Again, an accurate account will not be possible without specialist advice, but you can find out whether and how often the child walks to school and plays outdoor games. You can also find out how many hours a day the child spends watching television or playing on a computer. Information about the dietary habits and exercise patterns of other family members should also be taken; could the family afford and stick to a healthier diet if this were recommended?

Check also whether the obesity is causing any difficulties for the child such as being teased or causing low self-esteem. Is the child depressed? (See Section 7.7.) Does the child use food as a comfort? Is the child on regular medication?

Now, given the information you have obtained, try to understand how the weight problem has arisen in this particular child. Then go on to work out a plan to help.

### 6.2.3 Helping a child with obesity

Discuss with the child and family how they view the child's obesity. Then explain the dangers of obesity. If present, assess and treat type 2 diabetes or metabolic syndrome.

If the child and family wish to enter into a weight reduction programme, refer to a centre that has such programmes available. If this resource is not available, counsel along the following lines.

- Recommend a simple diet, containing locally available foods that will produce a calorie deficit. With children under the age of 5 years the parents should be able to control the child's intake relatively easily. With older children, explain that the whole family will need to go on this diet if it has any hope of success.
- Work out how the child can maintain the diet if he is eating away from home.
- Recommend a physical activity programme to take the place of some sedentary activities such as watching television and DVDs.
- Arrange for the child to be weighed regularly, praised and given small (non-food) rewards for any weight loss.
- If weight loss does occur, explain that relapse is likely and that the family need to be prepared to repeat the measures described above.

If the health professional is able to educate the local population on the risk of obesity, the following should be emphasised:

- breastfeeding of infants will lower the rates of later obesity
- from the earliest days children should receive diets that are healthy and have a low risk of producing excessive weight gain
- snacking between meals needs to be discouraged
- local schools should be encouraged to provide cheap, healthy school meals
- parents should be encouraged from the earliest days to limit the amount of time their children watch television and engage in other sedentary activities.

Now make a list of the ways in which the health professional might be able to help Alok.

## 6.3 Sleeping difficulties

**Case 6.3**

The mother of Ahmed, aged 2 years, an only child, was very embarrassed when she told the health professional what the problem was. Ahmed was a healthy child, developing normally and with nothing physically wrong with him. Nearly every night over the past year Ahmed has woken during the night. He has cried until either his mother or father have come to him in the next room. Then he goes back to sleep but wakes up half an hour later and cries again. It is very exhausting. She and her husband, Ahmed's father, were at their wits end when Ahmed went to a child minder. He spent quite a bit of time at the child minder's house asleep. It seemed a trivial problem but it was causing great tension between the parents. Ahmed's father blamed his wife because he thought she spoiled him and this was why he slept so badly. Both Ahmed's grandmothers thought his mother was useless because she could not control her child. The mother admitted she was quite depressed and getting to the end of her tether. She just did not know what to do and this silly problem was destroying her marriage. She was really guilty that she felt so angry with Ahmed.

### 6.3.1 Information about sleeping difficulties

**Children's sleep needs**

Children vary enormously in how much sleep they need. At 1 year of age, they sleep on average for 15 hours a day. By 2 years, they are sleeping an average of 13–14 hours, and by 4 years, an average of 12 hours. But this varies. A 4-year-old might easily manage on 8 hours or need as much as 15 hours. The amount a child needs does not always fit in with what the parents would like.

**Types of sleep problems**

The most frequent types of sleep problems in infancy and early childhood are unwillingness to go to bed or sleep and waking in the night. These are most common between 18 months and 4 years.

**Sleeping arrangements**

Sleep problems of this type are less common when there are traditional sleeping arrangements with all the family sleeping in one room. The child is less likely to feel anxious than if sleeping separately. If the family are all sleeping in the same room, the parents can comfort the waking child with little inconvenience to themselves. On the other hand, if a child is sleeping in the same room as the parents in a society where it is usual for children to sleep separately, this may indicate undue anxiety in the parents.

**Family influences**

In most cases, parents of children with sleep problems do not have significant mental health problems. Sometimes, for example, a mother's depression or anxiety or a father's alcohol problem may play a part. A sad, unhappy mother may really want to cling to her child during the night. An anxious mother may need to check that her baby is still breathing normally several times during the night. A father with an alcohol problem may arrive in the middle of the night and unsettle his wife and child by shouting or with violent behaviour.

## 6.3.2 How to find out more about a child with sleeping difficulties

- Find out what the sleeping arrangements are. Try to find out exactly what happens during the night. When does the child wake? What do the parents do? What happens then? If possible, get the parents to keep a diary for a week or so to establish exactly what is happening. If possible, try to get information from more than one family member.
- Assess family stresses and how they are affecting the situation.
- What have the parents tried so far?
- What do they think would be best to do next?

Now, given the information you have obtained, try to understand how the sleep problem has arisen in this particular child. Then go on to work out a plan to help.

## 6.3.3 How to help the parents with a child with sleeping difficulties

First, let the parents decide whether they think it is a good idea to take the child into their own bed. If the child is sleeping in a separate room, let the parents decide whether to keep the child in a separate room. Then work out a programme that will remove all reward from the child waking.

Second, establish a behavioural programme. For example, the parents may leave the child to cry. Eventually the child will stop. The child will then wake again but for a shorter period and then go back to sleep. This pattern will recur until the child barely wakes before going back to sleep. However, some parents will not be able to bring themselves to carry out such a programme. This approach is effective, but do not press parents to do something they really do not want to do. An alternative programme would be that when the child wakes, the parent goes into the room for the briefest moment and then leaves, even if the child cries. Either of these approaches can be combined with a star chart (Appendix 1). The child is rewarded with a star for desired behaviour such as going to bed without a fuss, or not calling for his parents when he wakes in the night. When the child has accumulated, for example, five stars, he can be rewarded with a small treat decided in advance. However, strongly discourage any reward for the child in waking, for example by having something to eat or drink. If the child is getting sweet drinks in the night, gradually replace with water and then no drink at all.

Finally, tell the mother that you do understand just how stressed she is. Agree it is not a small problem. Reassure her that the problem will almost certainly have stopped by the time the child is about 4 years old.

**Case 6.3** *(continued)*

When the health professional talked to Ahmed's mother it became clear that, apart from the sleep problem, there were no other stresses acting on the family. It turned out that she and her husband did not want Ahmed in their bed at night. However, they were rewarding him for waking up by giving him sweet drinks and telling him stories when he woke up. The health professional explained how this was encouraging Ahmed to wake up more. It was explained that the fact that he was getting so much sleep in the day meant he needed less sleep at night. The mother told the child minder to keep him active and not allow him more than 1 hour of sleep while he was with her. The mother agreed to reduce the amount of sweet drinks during the night and to gradually introduce water. She thought it was a good idea not to read him stories but just to go into the room briefly and settle him but not stay in the room even when he cried. Ahmed cried bitterly when he first realised that his parents were not going to stay in the room with him until he went to sleep, but they stayed firm. Gradually, Ahmed woke much less and cried less in the night, so that after 3 weeks the problem only happened very occasionally.

## 6.3.4 Prevention of sleep and waking problems in infants and young children

Parents should be encouraged:

- to help the child to feel safe and secure when going to bed and preparing for sleep
- to establish a regular bedtime
- to avoid exposing the child to overstimulating activities in the hour or so before bedtime, including watching scary movies or exciting television shows
- to develop a bedtime routine, for example with a regular wash before bed, a song or story for 10–15 minutes and then a firm 'Good-night' and departure from the room
- to establish a regular waking time before which they should be firm about returning the child to bed if he wakes early.

## 6.3.5 Sleep problems in later childhood and adolescence

As children develop, they need less sleep. The average 10-year-old sleeps for about 10 hours a night and the average 15- to 19-year-old, 7.5–8.5 hours. Adolescents occasionally complain of an inability to sleep (insomnia). They should be advised to follow these rules:

- have a regular waking-up time
- take a steady, daily amount of exercise
- make sure the bedroom is neither too hot nor too cold
- not to drink caffeine late in the evening
- not to smoke late in the evening (or even better, not to smoke at all)
- if not able to get to sleep because they are angry, frustrated or anxious, then they should not try harder and harder to fall asleep but get up and do something different, preferably in another room
- only go to bed when sleepy
- set the alarm and get up at the same time every morning regardless of how much they slept during the night
- not to nap during the day, if they are having difficulty sleeping at night.

In general, health professionals should avoid the use of hypnotic (sleep-inducing) drugs unless all the above measures have failed.

## 6.3.6 Other sleep problems

Note that all these sleep problems are likely to improve or disappear before or during adolescence, but just occasionally they do persist into adulthood.

### Nightmares

These are frightening dreams usually occurring in light sleep. The child or adolescent wakes in a frightened state and is able to remember the content of the dream. Usually this has to do with a frightening experience the evening or day before, such as a scary television programme, something the child has read or an event in school.

All children have occasional nightmares and, in this case, all that is needed is to give the child comfort and reassurance. Frequent nightmares (a couple of times a week or more) are a cause for concern and may be a sign of post-traumatic stress disorder (PTSD) (see pp. 168–170 for how to assess and what to do).

### Night terrors

These typically occur about 2 hours after the child (usually over 3 years but under 7 years old) has gone to sleep. The child sits up, utters a scream or shouts, moans and may walk around the house apparently unaware of the parents' presence. The child does not respond when spoken to or mutters a few muddled words. After a few minutes, but occasionally 20 minutes or more, the child returns to quiet sleep and has no recollection of the episode in the morning. Parents are often very frightened by these attacks but they are harmless and do not, in themselves, indicate emotional disturbance. They do not require any action. The parents should not try to wake the child. If the parents want to stop them and there is a regular pattern, they can try waking the child half hour or so before they occur and then let him go back to sleep.

### Sleep-walking and talking in sleep

The child or adolescent may sit up and then get up and walk about with a glazed expression. He may talk while doing this. After a few minutes he returns to his bed. Again he has no recollection of what has happened in the morning. No action needs to be taken. The child or adolescent should not be woken but may be gently guided back into bed. Because, extremely rarely, young people have been known to injure themselves in an episode of sleep-walking, sharp objects should be removed and all doors and windows should be locked at night to prevent them getting out.

### Obstructive sleep apnoea

This is a condition in which the child stops breathing for brief periods during sleep. The child snores loudly and has restless sleep. Most commonly this occurs because of the presence of large tonsils and adenoids. As a result of very brief periods when the brain is starved of oxygen, the condition may lead to a variety of behaviour and emotional problems, including irritability and attentional problems. If this condition is suspected, then, if at all possible, the child should be referred for further evaluation by a medically trained professional.

# 6.4 Bed-wetting

## 6.4.1 Information about bed-wetting

At birth and for some time afterwards, the bladder, empties automatically. By the age of 2 or 3 years most children can hold their urine in their bladder during the daytime until they get a feeling of fullness and empty their bladder. It takes longer for children to learn to hold their urine at night until they get up in the morning. Usually they manage this by the age of 3 or 4 years. By the age of 6–7 years, about 9 out of 10 children have stopped wetting the bed. Most who are still bed-wetting at that age will have stopped and be dry at night without treatment by the age of 10 years. Very few go on to wet the bed in adulthood. Most children who wet the bed at 7 years have never been dry. The technical term for wetting the bed is nocturnal enuresis.

### Case 6.4

Zoltan is a 7-year-old boy who is brought to a health clinic in the city by his very distressed mother because he is wetting the bed. Her three other children were all dry by day and night by the age of 3 years. Zoltan has only had three or four dry nights in the whole of his life. His mother has 'tried everything' to make him dry. She has shouted at him and told him he is behaving like a baby. She has made him wash his own sheets. Nothing has worked. She finds washing and cleaning the sheets every morning a great burden and expense. The family live in a tiny apartment and drying the sheets is a great problem. She has to go out to work for 9 hours a day and Zoltan just adds to her burdens. He seems to be doing well at school and has no other problems. She sometimes thinks he is sad and cries for no good reason, although he does not seem to care about the bed-wetting. Although his mother said she had no idea why Zoltan wet the bed, it turned out that she knew that both her husband and his brother had wet the bed until they were 10 years old.

## Causes of bed-wetting

As with all other areas of development there is wide variation in the age at which children gain bladder control. The age at which children gain bladder control is mainly inherited: some children are built to become dry early, others much later. Often one of the child's parents has been slow to become dry at night.

Children of mothers who punish or neglect their child may also gain bladder control later, although genetic influences are more important. If a child has a genetic tendency to wet the bed, the way mothers behave may tip the balance. In these cases there is an interaction between the genes and the environment.

Occasionally, stress may be an important factor in why a child wets the bed. This is most likely to be the case if the child has been dry for some months or years and then starts to wet the bed again. Bed-wetting may then continue even when the stress is no longer present.

Very occasionally, bed-wetting may be caused by illness, especially urinary infection or diabetes.

Delay in gaining bladder control may be one sign of general slowness of development (e.g. intellectual disability, see Chapter 5).

## Effects of bed-wetting

These will depend very much on the social circumstances in which the family is living. A child living in a hut in a poor rural area may be sleeping on the ground or on a mat. If the child wets himself at night, the urine will just seep away into the ground and no one will take much notice. A child who wets the bed while sleeping on a sheet over a mattress will, at the very least, give the mother more washing to do each day, which will be very hard for mothers to do if they are working. If there are servants to do the washing, this will not have as much impact.

## Effect on the child

Many children are ashamed of the fact that they wet the bed. They may think that they are the only ones to have this 'bad' habit. The fact that they wet the bed may, for example, mean they or their mothers think they cannot spend a night away from home at a friend's house. They may become sad and miserable, even depressed. If they become dry and their mood lifts, this suggests that the bed-wetting has been the cause of their low mood.

## Effect on the mother

Mothers often cannot decide whether they or their children are to blame for the bed-wetting. They may blame their child for not trying hard enough to become dry. The mother may think she has not brought her child up properly and feel guilty. So mothers change between being angry with the child and guilty about their own part in the problem. Some well-informed mothers will know that they have no need to blame themselves or their children – the wetting is just a sign of an isolated delay in development.

## Prevention

Healthcare professionals should encourage mothers of babies and infants not to worry too much about when their children become dry at night or stop wetting the bed. Most will gradually become dry first by day and then by night by the age of 5 years.

By day, mothers should praise their child at the first signs they want to use the toilet to pass urine. During the day mothers can remove nappies when the child is showing signs of being able to control his bladder. They should put them back on again if the child is clearly not ready. A dry night should be followed by praise but wet nights should not be punished. The mother should just remove the sheets without comment and replace them with clean ones.

## 6.4.2 Finding out more about a child who is wetting the bed

If the child is under the age of 5 or 6 years there is no need to enquire further unless there are other reasons for concern.

### For older children

- Obtain an account from the mother or both parents about the frequency with which the child wets the bed. Once or twice a night? Once a week or less?
- How does the mother react to the bed-wetting? Does she reward the child when he has a dry or drier night? Or does she punish the child for wetting the bed?
- Is there any evidence that the child has a physical problem causing the bed-wetting? This would be very unusual, but needs checking. Does the child have pain passing urine? Has the child had any blood in the urine? How often does the child pass urine in the daytime? Is the child dry by day?

- Rule out diabetes or urinary infection by testing the urine.
- Find out what the parents have already tried, including restricting fluids before bedtime, lifting the child during the night, etc.
- What effect is the bed-wetting having on the everyday lives of the child and the mother?

Now, given the information you have obtained, try to understand how the bed-wetting has arisen in this particular child. Then go on to work out a plan to help.

## 6.4.3 Helping children who are wetting the bed

With children who are wetting the bed under the age of 6 years, the mother should be reassured that this is quite normal and that probably the child will gain control within the next year or two. She should avoid punishing the child.

### Children over the age of 6 years

- In children who have been wet from birth, check to find out whether there is evidence of developmental delay or intellectual disability (see Chapters 4 and 5).
- In children who have been dry but have then started to wet the bed again, ask whether there are any stresses acting on the child. If stresses are present, try to work out ways with the mother and child of reducing or eliminating these.
- In children who do not have any physical problem, reassure the parents and child. Explain that this is a very common problem and is extremely likely to get better over the next year or so.
- Encourage the parents not to give too much attention to the problem. Parents should reward success without drawing attention to failure.
- Strongly discourage emotional (insulting, teasing) or physical punishment for bed-wetting.
- Discourage giving the child a lot of drinks during the evening and night both before and after the child goes to bed.
- Encourage the child to go to the toilet before going to bed.
- Suggest to the parents they might try to wake the child up before they go to bed themselves for the night. If they have learned when the bed-wetting takes place in the night, they might try to wake the child just before this time and encourage him to empty his bladder.
- Try the use of a star chart (Appendix 1) to encourage dryness by rewarding the child for dry nights. A star is stuck onto the chart the morning after the child has a dry night. When the child has accumulated an agreed number of stars, the child is given a small treat. No comment is made about nights when the child wets the bed, but the child does not get a star for those nights. Such a chart is used to emphasise achievement. It also provides a baseline for the problem and can form a record of the child's progress. In about a quarter of cases, it will produce some definite improvement.
- Bladder training may be useful if the child is wetting in the daytime. Parents encourage the child to wait slightly longer each time between passing urine. They can do this by encouraging the child to try to wait for at least a few minutes when the bladder is full, before he empties it.
- In high-income countries, a variety of alarms are available to try to deal with this problem when it occurs in older children.
- Wetting the bed at night is, in itself, not an indication for a talking treatment (see p. 7). However, children and parents do benefit when health professionals explain sympathetically why a child is wetting the bed. If the child is anxious or depressed in addition to wetting the bed, then a talking treatment should be used (see Section 2.3.1).

- Regarding medication, a tricyclic antidepressant may be helpful if it is particularly important for a child to be dry over two or three nights, for example if the child is going away with his class for a trip or is spending a night or two at a friend's home. Imipramine (25 mg) can be used for short-term situations but should not be used long term. In parts of the world where it is available, desmopressin, either as a nasal spray or tablets, may be used.
- With the very small number of children who continue to wet the bed into adolescence and even adulthood, make sure they are not punished. They may need help to be able to explain to boyfriends/girlfriends what the matter with them is.

Now describe how the health professional might be able to help Zoltan.

# 6.5 Soiling

**Case 6.5**
Nikhil is a 7-year-old boy brought by his mother to the clinic in the city because he is soiling his underwear. He was clean and dry by the age of 3 years. Then, shortly after he started school at the age of 6 years, he began to come home with faeces in his underwear. To begin with there was just slight soiling and his mother did not say anything about it. But, after a few weeks, he began to pass whole motions into his underwear. Other children complained of the smell and tried to avoid sitting near him but Nikhil did not seem to notice the smell. His mother told him to stop and after she had changed him when he came home from school she punished him by not letting him go out to play. But this did not make any difference. What should the health professional advise?

## 6.5.1 Information about soiling
### Control of the bowels
Normally, children first show interest in passing their motions into a pot between the ages of 18 months and 2 years. On average, bowel control is achieved by the age of about 2.5 or 3 years, but it is not unusual or abnormal for this to be delayed until about 4 years.

Mostly, bowel control comes about because the child is physiologically ready. The process is helped along if the parents encourage and praise steps in the right direction. The process will be delayed or go wrong if parents punish a child for not performing in the right way. Delay beyond the age of 4 years may be linked to intellectual disability. Delay in obtaining bowel control also tends to run in families and thus might be due to genetic influences.

Soiling over the age of 4 years is caused by constipation or difficulty in passing faeces (unusually hard) with overflow – this is easily the most common reason for soiling. Occasionally there is encopresis – the passing of normal faeces in inappropriate places. There may also be a mixture of the above two.

### Constipation with overflow of soft/liquid faeces
A constipated child passes hard faeces into the pot or toilet pan but liquid faeces accumulating above the constipated mass may leak out and cause liquid soiling.

Chronic constipation usually starts in infancy but may begin later, for example after an episode of anal fissure when defecation has been painful. After a prolonged period of constipation the bowel becomes stretched and the child can lose the normal sensation of the need to pass faeces.

If the problem has been present from birth and the child has always been badly constipated, with no period without constipation, there may be a serious physical problem affecting the nervous supply to the lower part of the bowel and, if possible, the child needs to see a specialist. Usually constipation arises because of:

- excessive attempts by the mother to 'train' the child too early and to administer punishment if he does not 'perform'. In contrast, control of the bowel may also fail to develop because the child is being brought up in neglectful circumstances with no training and nobody minding too much if he soils or not;
- a diet lacking in fibre, with adequate fruit and vegetables and plenty of water to drink;
- stressful family circumstances;
- fear of using the toilet. This may occur after an episode of painful constipation or, in an anxious child, after an upsetting experience or because the child has frightening fantasies, for example, of being bitten by something in the toilet;
- a child who has learned he can 'control' his parents by withholding faeces;
- sexual abuse. The child may have been hurt in this way and be frightened that passing a motion will cause pain. This is an unusual cause.

**Passing normal motions in inappropriate places (encopresis)**

- This is uncommon.
- This may be present from birth or there may have been a period when the child was clean but soiling recurred after a stressful experience.
- Mild constipation may be present, making things worse.
- It may occur at school or the child may only pass a motion on the way home from school.
- The child may go to some lengths to hide his dirty clothes.
- The child may smear his faeces on the walls or over furniture. This is likely to be a sign that the child feels aggressive towards his parents.
- Children with encopresis often show other behaviour or emotional problems, especially aggressive behaviour at home and elsewhere.
- The child might also have significant learning problems.

## 6.5.2 Finding out more about a child who is soiling

The health professional first needs to find out from the mother and child the following.

- How and when, if at all, did the child develop bowel continence, become clean and able to go to the toilet to pass motions?
- What sort of training, if any, did the parents use? Is there any suggestion the mother found contact with the child's faeces distasteful or repugnant?
- If the child was clean and then lost bowel control, what was happening at the time that might have been upsetting for the child?
- Is the child frightened of using the toilet?
- Has anyone else in the family, parents or brothers and sisters, been slow to establish bowel control?
- What is the child's diet like? Does it contain enough roughage, i.e. fruit, vegetables, liquids?
- What is the consistency of the motions that are passed? In particular, are they normal in consistency or unusually hard/liquid, or a mixture of hard and liquid?
- What is the child's attitude to the soiling? Is he upset about it or not seem to mind?
- Does the child use the faeces in any way, for example, smear them around?
- What are relationships in the family like? Do family members generally get on well or is there a good deal of shouting and arguments?
- How is the child getting on at school? Is he making progress? Is there any evidence that he is a bully or is bullied himself?

- Does he have any other behaviour, learning or emotional problems?

After obtaining an account of the problem, the health professional should carry out a physical examination, looking especially for:

- a distended, swollen abdomen
- faecal masses that can be felt in the abdomen or by rectal examination
- any evidence of disease or trauma in the anal region – the scars of a fissure may be present or there may be evidence of trauma suggestive of sexual abuse.

If indicated, an X-ray of the abdomen should be carried out to detect faecal masses. No other radiological investigation is necessary.

Now, given the information you have obtained, try to understand how the soiling has arisen in this particular child. Then go on to work out a plan to help.

## 6.5.3 Helping a child who is soiling

Where there is any evidence of constipation, the first priority is to empty the bowel using the following procedure.

The child should be given oral laxatives. Most children, but not all, will respond. If the laxative medication fails to have sufficient effect, the child should be given an enema. Once the bowel is cleared out, the child should be put on a maintenance laxative as it may be many months before the bowel regains the capacity to function without such medication.

The child's diet should be considered and the parents encouraged to provide a high-fibre diet with a good fluid intake. At the same time the parents should be strongly encouraged to establish regular visits to the toilet with rewards for going to the toilet, a bigger reward for attempting to pass a motion and an even bigger reward for actually passing a motion. This procedure should be recorded on a star chart (Appendix 1).

Both children and parents should be given clear explanations about how the bowel functions so that they can become more self-reliant in this area.

If the constipation continues after all these measures have been taken, try to refer for a more specialist opinion as there are other rare causes of constipation.

When there is no evidence of constipation but there is soiling, then the physical process of normal defecation should be described to the child and parents so that they understand what is happening.

A routine of regular visits to the toilet should be established. The child should again be rewarded for going to the toilet, given a slightly bigger reward for trying and an even bigger reward if he is successful in passing a motion in the toilet. This should be accompanied by the show of a good deal of positive affection towards the child and a star chart system, recording success (Appendix 1), should be established.

The child should be given the opportunity to express his feelings about his family members. Good questions to ask are: 'A lot of children I see get very cross with their mum or dad. Does that ever happen to you?' and 'What sort of things make you angry?' If the health professional feels confident about such an approach, she can undertake a small number of family interviews in which the child and parents can express to each other their feelings about the soiling and other family matters. It is important that the health professional does not take sides even if she feels very strongly that either the parents or the child are in the right. In most cases this approach will be moderately successful and the child's soiling will be reduced or even disappear altogether. Soiling in adulthood is very unusual but it does occur.

If constipation persists, there may be a number of rare conditions present and, if possible, the child should be referred for further investigation.

## 6.6 Tics and other jerky movements

**Case 6.6**

Aadi is a 7-year-old boy whose mother brought him to the clinic because he keeps blinking his eyes. He also has some twitching of other parts of his face. This started about a year ago but has become worse in the past 2 months. When his mother tells him to stop, it just seems to make him do it more. It is also worse when he has work at school that he finds hard. His mother is very cross with him because she knows he can stop this blinking if he wants to. He is also restless and overactive and has poor attention and concentration. He is an only child. His father would have liked to have come along, but cannot take time off work. He has an office job and often works late in the evening as he is so conscientious. What should the health professional do?

### 6.6.1 Information about tics and other jerky movements

Tics are rapid, repeated movements such as blinking or twitching of the face. Usually, it is only the face that is affected, but sometimes other parts of the body are involved. Children who are seriously affected may show quite violent, sudden movements of the arms or legs. Involuntary sounds, voices or noises such as throat-clearing, grunts and even brief screams or shouts may occur. When several movement (motor) tics and at least one sound (vocal) tic have been present for more than a year, the condition is known as Tourette syndrome.

Tics of the face usually begin round about the age of 5 or 6 years. They may be made worse by anxiety, stress or boredom. Some types of tics disappear after a few weeks, while other types persist. If people draw attention to them or children are told off or asked to stop, the tics usually get worse. They may be less prominent when the child is occupied or relaxed. One type of movement may get replaced by a new one over time.

The more severe form, Tourette syndrome, is often linked to problems of attention and concentration (see Section 8.2), obsessions and compulsions (see Section 7.8), and sleep difficulties. Very occasionally there may be involuntary swearing (coprolalia). In addition, there may be other family members with tics or obsessions and compulsions. Genetic influences are important.

### 6.6.2 Finding out more about children with tics and other jerky movements

Find out when the problem began, what parts of the body it affects, what makes it better or worse, and what the parents and child think have caused it. Are there any particular stresses that seem to bring the tics on?

Check for the presence of other problems, such as difficulties in attention or hyperactivity (see Section 8.2) and obsessions and compulsions (see Section 7.8), or self-injurious behaviours. Ask whether other members of the family have had the same sort of problem.

Now, given the information you have obtained, try to understand how the tics have arisen in this particular child. Then go on to work out a plan to help.

### 6.6.3 Helping children with tics and other jerky movements

Explain to the parents and child that the tics are outside the child's control. He really cannot help these sudden movements.

Having identified any stresses that seem to be making the problem worse, see how far they can be removed. In addition, help the child to be more aware of what brings the tics on. More information on awareness training and other specific behavioural techniques for managing tics can be found at www.cdc.gov/ncbddd/tourette/treatments.html.

Medication can be effective but is not needed if there are only a few tics and these are not causing any serious problems. For severe tics (Tourette syndrome), it is worthwhile considering medication. Clonidine (see Appendix 2) can be used if tics and hyperactivity are both present. A very small dose of haloperidol or risperidone (see Appendix 2) can also help control the tics. The dose can be increased slowly if side-effects do not occur. Side-effects to look out for are drowsiness and, most alarming, muscle spasms producing a twisted posture (dystonic reactions). Stop the medication immediately if muscle spasms occur. Associated problems such as difficulties with attention, hyperactivity or obsessions and compulsions will need appropriate treatment (see the relevant sections).

Now make a list of the ways in which the health professional might be able to help Aadi.

# CHAPTER 7

# Emotional problems

Emotional problems may involve:

- excessive worrying, fear and anxiety: sometimes the fears may be focused on specific objects or situations, sometimes the anxiety may be more general. Refusal to go to school often arises from anxiety;
- excessive misery, unhappiness and depression: usually low mood is linked to a loss or other stress, but sometimes lowering of mood may appear without obvious cause. Particularly worrying features of depression are ideas of self-harming as well as acts of self-harm that may indeed be fatal;
- compulsions and obsessions: these may involve the need to check everything far more often than is necessary or carry out time-consuming rituals.

## 7.1 Introduction to anxiety problems

### 7.1.1 Information about anxiety problems

Anxiety is a normal human emotion. It occurs when we are faced with a real or imagined danger. It is an unpleasant sensation which we want to stop. We make it stop by dealing with the danger or by removing ourselves from the scene. We may also realise that the danger is only imaginary and there is nothing to worry about. Anxiety is necessary for us to survive as it warns us about danger and thus protects us from it.

Anxiety may present with physical symptoms such as tiredness or headaches, and mental symptoms such as irritability, inability to relax and 'feeling on edge'. It may also present with physical or mental signs of a panic attack (see Section 7.2).

Sometimes children and adolescents experience too much anxiety which stops them from leading a normal life. When this happens they are in need of help. There are various types of excessive anxiety:

- panic attacks (see Section 7.2)
- phobias (see Section 7.3)
- school refusal (see Section 7.4)
- separation problems (see Section 7.5)
- excessive shyness (see Section 7.6).

In addition, sometimes children and adolescents feel anxious generally. Examples include:

- worries about how good they are at school or at a particular sport, about examinations or sporting competitions
- excessive self-consciousness and the need for reassurance

- restlessness, nervousness, inability to relax
- physical symptoms, such as tension, light-headedness, heart beating fast, stomach discomfort and dizziness when there is no physical reason why these should be present
- difficulty concentrating
- irritability.

Usually general anxiety occurs because children have an inborn tendency to be more worried and anxious. Often, but not always, they have anxious, worrying parents. Such parents have inherited a tendency to be anxious from their parents. In addition, because their parents worry about them, they worry about themselves. However, it is not always parents who make children anxious. It must be remembered that children who worry can make their parents anxious.

Ways of finding out more about generally anxious children and helping them can be found by consulting the other sections in this chapter which deal with specific anxiety problems. Helpful interventions include yoga and breathing and relaxation exercises (see below) and anxiety management strategies including cognitive–behavioural therapy (CBT) (see p. 7). The most common ways of helping children with anxiety are:

- listening and talking to them and their parents
- trying to find ways of giving them the skills to deal with their excessive fears
- changing the situations that appear to make them anxious
- breathing exercises and relaxation techniques.

### Breathing exercises

Teach the child to breathe in slowly through the nose, and out through the mouth. Children should breathe in and count up to 5 while holding the air in and then breathe out while counting up to 5 (breathing in, two, three, four, five, and out, two, three, four, five – at a rate of about one count per second). Adolescents could count up to 10 while breathing in and out. Similarly, for abdominal breathing exercises the child is asked to notice that the abdominal wall goes out when taking air in and goes in when breathing out.

### Muscle relaxation

Young children may find it easier to start with a visual imagery. Have the child close their eyes and imagine a relaxing place of their choice such as a garden, beach, park, playing with a favourite person or pet. Once the child has chosen a place and while the child is imagining this, describe the place to them, including what they might see, hear, feel and smell. Younger children may use a picture or drawing to help them in the beginning. The child is then taught to tense and relax major groups of muscles in a fixed order. Train the child to tense or tighten a group of muscles, feel the tension by holding it tight and then gradually relax. This training usually starts with the muscles of the forehead, then the shoulders and upper limbs, then the chest and abdomen, and finally the legs and toes. Audiotapes and CDs are also available to help children learn and practice relaxation techniques.

### Medication

Medication – in particular, where they are available, low doses of selective serotonin reuptake inhibitors – can be helpful in some children and adolescents. Short courses of anxiolytic medication may also be useful. But medication, especially anxiolytic medication, should be used with caution as there is always a risk that children may become drug-dependent. It may be very difficult to stop medication for anxiety once it has been started. See Appendix 2 for medication that may be used in anxiety disorders.

## 7.2 Panic attacks

**Case 7.1**

Ahan is a 15-year-old boy whose father brought him to a health professional because of a fear that he had something wrong with his heart. He had six panic attacks which occurred suddenly, without warning. They all occurred when he was leaving the house to spend the evening with his friend, Alok. He would walk a few steps and then find his heart beating very fast. Someone had told him how to feel his pulse and it was really racing. He felt panic-stricken. His legs felt weak and he thought he would collapse but he managed to stagger home. There did not seem to be any reason for these attacks. His parents really liked Alok, who had an older, very beautiful 16-year-old sister. Sometimes his parents even thought they might arrange a marriage between Ahan and this girl, whose family they respected.

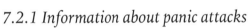

### *7.2.1 Information about panic attacks*

These are attacks of extreme anxiety, sometimes coming on without warning. At other times they occur before a situation of which the child or adolescent is very frightened. The physical signs of a panic attack are:

- rapid beating of the heart, with palpitations
- breathlessness and tightness in the chest
- dizziness
- 'butterflies' or even pain in the stomach
- a weak feeling in the legs.

The mental signs of a panic attack are:

- intolerable anxiety or tension
- fear of dying
- fear of going mad
- fear of losing control.

The child or adolescent may not be aware of the reasons why he is getting such attacks. By talking about when the attacks occur it may become possible to understand what the child or adolescent is so anxious about.

### *7.2.2 Finding out more about a child or adolescent with panic attacks*

- Find out how long these attacks have been going on.
- Has the child had panic attacks before?
- What seems to bring them on – situations which he is worried about (examinations, arguments with a friend, parents getting ill or going away), relationship difficulties, etc.?
- Possible toxic effects of coffee, caffeine-containing fizzy drinks?
- Examine the child to make sure that there is no underlying physical cause.

- Carry out any relevant physical tests: blood pressure and pulse – rate and regularity. An electrocardiogram might be indicated if the equipment is available.

Now, given the information you have obtained, try to understand how the panic attacks have arisen in this particular child. Then go on to work out a plan to help.

### 7.2.3 Helping children and adolescents with panic attacks

Deal with any physical problems. If physical problems have been ruled out, then you should:

- sit the child or adolescent down calmly
- reassure him that he does not have a physical illness
- tell him that he is not going to die or go mad
- if relevant, tell him that he is not under a spell or been bewitched
- tell him that he will feel better shortly
- if he is breathing too fast, help him to breathe more slowly in a steady manner.

Once the panic attack has stopped:

- try to deal with any stresses that may have precipitated the attack
- work out with the child or adolescent how he can avoid having a panic attack if the same situation arises in the future. For example, if acutely stressed, it can be suggested that he calls a friend or a parent, use relaxation exercises, listens to some music, etc., until he is feeling better.
- practice deep breathing and relaxation exercises (see p. 53). Cognitive–behavioural therapy (see p. 7) can also be useful.

Medication may be helpful occasionally in severe cases (see Appendix 2).

Now make a list of the ways in which the health professional might be able to help Ahan.

## 7.3 Fears and phobias

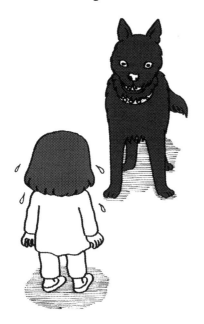

**Case 7.2**

Yoko is a 4-year-old girl who has always been a bit fearful. About a week ago she was shopping with her mother in the market buying fruit and vegetables when a large black dog snarled at her and then started to bark. The dog was held by a strong lead, but the stall-holder who owned the dog pretended to untie the lead to frighten Yoko more. He laughed at her. Yoko was petrified. Now she has been brought to the health professional by her mother because she will not go out of the house in case she meets the dog again. She is sleeping poorly and has nightmares of being bitten by the dog. Her mother is at her wits end and does not know what to do.

### 7.3.1 Information about specific fears (animals, strangers, the dark, thunderstorms)

In the early years, between 2 and 5 years, children are likely to be frightened by the unusual or the unexpected. Phobias (disabling fears) of animals (e.g. spiders, dogs, mice), of the dark, and of strangers are very common. It is only when the phobia lasts more than a few days and stops the child carrying out everyday activities that there is a need for help. The phobia is usually triggered by a single unpleasant experience, but there may be repeated unpleasant experiences. Specific phobias nearly always disappear over a few days or weeks without treatment but they are very unpleasant while they last, so if one can do anything to shorten them this is well worth doing. Boys and girls are equally affected, although children who have anxious personalities are more likely to be affected.

Some children when they enter school are too frightened to speak there even though they speak normally at home. These are said to have selective mutism – a phobia of speaking.

### 7.3.2 Finding out more about children with specific fears

The health professional should listen to the parent's story, asking questions about when the phobia began, what started it, how it is affecting the child's life, whether it is getting better by itself, whether the child's sleep is affected and what the parent has done to make the child better. Usually the diagnosis of a specific phobia is a straightforward matter. There is usually no need to do a physical examination unless there are indicators in the story to suggest this might be helpful.

Now, given the information you have obtained, try to understand how the phobia has arisen in this particular child. Then go on to work out a plan to help.

### 7.3.3 Helping children with specific fears

If the phobia is already reducing in intensity, there is no need to take any action other than to reassure the mother that it will get better. If it has persisted for more than a month, then the health professional should give active advice to the mother and suggest an approach called desensitisation. This involves very gradual introduction to the feared object or situation until the child can be exposed to it with confidence. The mother should be able to manage this by herself if the health professional can give clear instructions along the following lines. The mother (or father, but usually it will be the mother) should:

- make a list of all the things the child is afraid of, starting with the least frightening and continuing to the most frightening – she should do this with the child;
- she should then work out with the child how she is going to manage the task of overcoming the least frightening situation;
- the child should get a lot of praise, kisses, cuddles and perhaps a small reward such as a sweet for having managed this least frightening task;
- once the child is able to perform this least frightening task with confidence, the next most frightening task should be tackled in the same way;
- this process should continue until the child is able to lead a normal life.

Now describe how the health professional might be able to help Yoko.

In fact, this is what happened. As suggested, the mother talked to the child about the problem and together they composed a list from the least frightening to the most frightening situation.

1   Looking out of a closed window and being able to look at a dog without drawing back
2   Doing the same through an open window
3   Standing at the front door (porch) for 5 minutes with her mother
4   Going for a walk of about 100 yards up the road with her mother, on the understanding that if a dog appeared they would cross the road
5   As above but on the understanding that if a dog came the other way they would walk past the dog
6   Going for longer walks along the same lines
7   Revisiting the market but keeping clear of the dog that had frightened Yoko
8   Going towards the frightening dog but keeping a few feet away

The mother then took Yoko slowly through the above steps, making sure she felt secure before going on to the next step. When Yoko had successfully completed the last step, the treatment was seen as finished.

## 7.4 Refusal to go to school

**Case 7.3**

Bindar is a 10-year-old boy who is brought to the health professional because he will not go to school. This began about 6 months ago. He was at first reluctant to go to school and kept making excuses why he should not go. He complained of headaches, and also said that boys were picking on him on his way to school. Three months ago he refused to go at all. He has been spending the time at home playing, going with his mother to her workplace and watching television. His mother and father (a rather quiet man, not very forceful), have tried to get him back to school, but without success. Because of the headaches, the health professional examined Bindar but found no physical problem with him. She talked a bit more to his mother. It turned out that when the problem with school began, his mother was depressed because her own mother had died. Also at this time, a male teacher of whom Bindar was rather frightened had shouted at him for talking when he should have been paying attention. Bindar has always been a rather sensitive boy and was very upset, saying that he thought this teacher might beat him.

### 7.4.1 Information about children who refuse to go to school

There are three main reasons why children will not go to school.

1   Separation anxiety (see Section 7.5). In these situations children refuse to go because of fear of separation. They may be worried about something bad happening to their parent when they are away at school or of being abandoned by them.
2   A fear of something happening in school (e.g. bullying) or of a person (e.g. teacher). If a child will not go to school for either of these reasons, the parents know about it from their own observations or from the school.
3   A dislike of school, with a wish to get involved in other, often antisocial, activities. This reason for not attending school is truancy. In this situation the parents do not know about their child's non-attendance at school (see Section 8.7).

Sometimes children will not go to school because of a combination of the first two points, for example they may hate to leave their parents and also are frightened of being bullied in school.

## 7.4.2 Finding out more about a child who will not go to school

- Obtain an account of how the problem has developed and what it consists of from the mother.
- It is likely that the mother will have brought the child to the clinic with a physical complaint such as a headache, stomach ache or joint pains. Examine the child to rule out any physical problem causing these physical symptoms.
- Talk, if possible, to both parents about the problem. Try to understand how they see it. Ask questions such as 'Why do you think X is having such difficulty getting to school?' Your approach will be very different depending on whether they think he has a physical illness or understand that he is too anxious to attend.
- If there are two parents in the home, see whether they view the problem in the same way. This will be easier if the health professional can manage to see them both: if this is not possible the health professional can ask the mother what her husband thinks about the problem.
- Find out from the parents about how the child is spending the time when he is not at school. Do they give him jobs or schoolwork to do or is he left to please himself?
- Find out what they have already done to get their child back to school. Have they spoken to his teacher about it?
- Find out about the possible reasons why the child will not go to school. His fearfulness may be related to his home life or with school or with both.
- Ask especially about the mother's physical and mental health. Might the child be worried about her because she has a physical illness? Or is she, like Bindar's mother, unusually depressed or anxious?
- Remember that anxiety about separation involves two people: the child and the person the child is anxious about separating from. It is much more difficult for a child to separate from a mother who is worried about separating from him than from a mother who really wants her child to become as independent as other children of the same age. You can ask questions such as 'How do you feel when X is at home. Some mothers feel more settled when they have their children at home and they can see what they are up to. Do you feel like that?' or 'Some mothers feel so low they find it easier if they have someone with them during the day. Do you feel like that with X?'
- Listen and talk to the child. If possible, it is better to see the child separately, but because of time constraints or because the child refuses to be separated from his parent this may not be possible. If this is the case it is still possible to listen and talk to the child with his parent(s) present.
- This may be difficult, but if at all possible, talk to the child's teacher or head teacher about the problem. The amount of interest schools take in this sort of problem varies greatly. In some schools the teachers will have noticed that the child is absent and be very keen to help in any way they can. In other schools, the teachers may be so overwhelmed with the numbers of children they have to teach that they may not notice the absence or may even be quite relieved to have one less student, even if this is a child not causing any problems, like Bindar. It is important to try to find out how the school sees the problem and what time and effort they might be able to put into resolving it.

Now, given the information you have obtained, try to understand how the refusal to go to school has arisen in this particular child. Then go on to work out a plan to help.

## 7.4.3 Helping a child who refuses to go to school

Once a health professional has obtained information as described above, it should be a relatively straightforward matter to work out an action plan. This will involve:

- reducing the stresses preventing the child getting back to school, and
- insisting that he starts to attend school again on a regular basis as soon as possible.

This might mean talking to the school, parents and child.

### Talking to the school

Is the school willing to have the child back in school? If he goes back to school, would the school be prepared to try to make life as easy as possible for him in the first few days until he is used to attending again. How does the school suggest this might be done: spending time with the school secretary, making sure that all teachers know how hard it has been for Bindar to attend school? Would a local teacher have time to pick Bindar up from his home? Or are there other students in the neighbourhood that Bindar can go to school with?

### Talking to the parents

Explain to the mother how her need to have the child at home with her is preventing him from going back. Does she think she could manage if he was not at home but attending school regularly? Could she try not to take the child to work with her but make some other arrangements that would be less attractive for him? Could she make sure that he is not rewarded for not attending school by not making life so easy for him when he is absent, for example by insisting he has no television or computer games during school hours? She could try to ensure he does continue to see his friends after school hours. Is she depressed? If so, could she be treated for her depressive disorder? Could she get a course of antidepressants for herself?

Talk to the father about how he might help to get the child back to school. Could he be involved in taking him? Would this be helpful?

### Talking to the child

Make sure he understands how important it is for him and his future that he goes back to school. Tell him there is really no alternative – and that everyone is in agreement that he has to return to school. It is important to give him the opportunity to confide what is upsetting him. Ask him what he thinks would be helpful.

Then with both parents and the child present, work out when the child will go back to school. Try to do this with confidence, not even allowing the suggestion that he is not going to make it, although admitting it is not going to be easy for him or his parents. Hopefully it will have been possible to enlist the help of the school. The child being greeted at the gate by a friend or a helpful member of the school staff can help reduce the anxiety.

### Severe cases

A step-by-step approach may be needed in severe cases where the child spends gradually increasing periods of time at school. If he feels overwhelmed or panicky while at school, he should be supported and allowed to spend time away from the classroom in a quiet place such as the library until he calms down. In most cases this approach will be successful in getting a child back into school. But it is important for the parents to keep the pressure up because if the child starts taking the occasional day off, this can rapidly result in a recurrence of school refusal.

In cases where there is significant anxiety or panic symptoms, this will need to be addressed and managed appropriately (see Section 7.2).

It is likely that the child will remain an anxious boy. His parents will need to remain firm with him when he shows signs of falling back into bad habits, but he should be able to lead a normal life in the future.

Now make a list of the ways in which the health professional might be able to help Bindar.

## 7.5 Separation anxiety

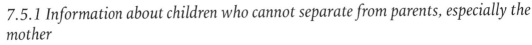

**Case 7.4**

Serena is a 4-year-old girl who is brought to the health professional in a city clinic because for the past 2 years she will not go anywhere without her mother. Her father has never lived with her mother and she does not see him. She developed normally until about the age of 2 years when her mother had to go into hospital for 3 months because of tuberculosis. While her mother was in hospital, Serena was looked after by an aunt who already had six children and who could not really cope with another child. Serena was ignored, not given enough to eat, teased and bullied by the older children, and frequently punished for very minor disobedience. Her mother responded well to treatment and when she came out of hospital she was able to look after Serena again. But as soon as she was reunited with her, Serena would not allow her mother to leave her sight. She insisted on sleeping with her. Her mother needed to go to work but Serena would scream and scream if she attempted to leave her with a babysitter. The health professional examined Serena but found nothing physically the matter with her.

### 7.5.1 Information about children who cannot separate from parents, especially the mother

Children normally go through a period of anxiety when they are separated from their mother. This period of separation begins in the first year of life, but is at its height between 18 months and 4 years (see Chapter 15). It may persist throughout life.

The way children show separation anxiety varies depending on their family lives. Some children are brought up by their mother only; others have many people responsible for their care, including grandparents, aunts, uncles, older brothers and sisters. A child is more likely to have separation anxiety problems if brought up by just one or two people. This is less likely to happen in LAMI countries than in high-income countries.

In some children, this period of normal separation anxiety may become so acute that the child is seriously troubled. If the child is over 4 years old there will be a need for the health professional to help. The mother and child may need assistance if there is presence of:

- unrealistic and persistent worry about harm happening to attachment figures, especially parents, of whom the child is very fond, leading to a fear that they will leave and not return
- persistent reluctance or refusal to leave the home, for example, to go to school so as to not be separated from attachment figures (see Chapter 15)
- persistent reluctance or refusal to go to sleep without being near an attachment figure or to go to sleep away from home – this is not relevant if the child and parent(s) normally sleep in the same room
- repeated nightmares involving the theme of separation
- excessive distress (anxiety, crying, tantrums, apathy, withdrawal) regarding separation
- presence of physical symptoms such as frequent headache, stomach ache, nausea or vomiting arising from fear of separation.

The child may have unusual problems in separating because:

- the mother is communicating her anxiety about being apart.
- the child has been ill treated (see Sections 14.3–14.6) and is frightened of this happening again if parted from his mother
- the child is threatened with the mother or father leaving home if he is naughty – children are sometimes told they will be given away if they are naughty.
- the child is temperamentally very anxious – he has inherited a tendency to be anxious
- a mixture of the above.

The child's problem in separating is likely to link with the mother's anxiety about being apart from her child. This may show itself by:

- the mother being a generally anxious person
- the mother finding it very hard to be apart because, for example:
  - this child is very special to her because she had difficulty becoming pregnant or because the child was very ill at birth or is the youngest
  - she knows the child has been ill-treated and feels guilty about it
  - she is frightened of her mother or mother-in-law who thinks she is no good at looking after her child, so she has to be especially protective and not let the child out of her sight.

## 7.5.2 Finding out more about children who have unusual difficulty separating

Find out whether the child's degree of anxiety is greater than one would normally expect in a child of this age in the community in which the family is living. To do this, obtain a story from the mother or both parents about the nature of the child's problem in separating. Check for the presence of any of the problems described above. All these are reasons the child and mother may need help.

If the child is unusually anxious in situations of separation, check for possible reasons the child may have a tendency to be anxious (see above). Also, check for possible reasons the mother may find it difficult to be apart from her child (see above). But remember, the mother may not be anxious about separating; she may just have a very anxious child. Remember too that some children are so anxious that they make their mothers anxious. Check for any signs of the child being ill-treated or whether he has been ill treated in the past (see Sections 14.3–14.6). Find out how the mother is dealing with the situation at the present time. Is she using threats or providing reassurance?

Observe how the child responds to his mother while they are both in front of you. Can the child even go to another part of the room to do a drawing? Or is the child unusually clingy? Remember though, many children are unusually anxious when a stranger approaches them. The child's behaviour with you may not be typical of how he usually behaves.

Now, given the information you have obtained, try to understand how the separation anxiety has arisen in this particular child. Then go on to work out a plan to help.

### 7.5.3 Helping children who have unusual difficulty separating

- If a child is having unusual difficulty separating, discuss with the mother how she sees the problem. Does she think the child's behaviour is unusual?
- What does she think the cause of the problem might be?
- What has she already done about it? Is she reassuring and does she cuddle the child if he is anxious? Or does she threaten him that she will leave or that she will give him away?
- You can take various steps to help a child and mother when a child has unusual difficulty separating. You can:
  - encourage the mother to use reassurance rather than threats of punishment
  - talk with the child about what he is frightened of during a period of separation
  - try and work out ways in which the mother can get other people involved in looking after the child with her; this will result in the child depending less on her and more on other people
  - gradually increase the time she can be away from her child; she can start with a separation of just a few seconds and gradually lengthen this by a few minutes at a time
  - make sure the child has interesting things to do when she is separated from him.

Now describe how the health professional might be able to help Serena.

## 7.6 Excessive shyness

**Case 7.5**
Amrita is a 14-year-old girl brought by her mother to the health professional because she has a mole on her face. The mole is really quite small and the health professional cannot see what the fuss is all about. Is there any other problem? It turns out that Amrita has dizzy spells. It is clear that these occur because she does not want to go out to mix with other girls in their homes. She can see one girl at a time, and indeed she has one good friend, but when it comes to little groups of girls she says she does not want to go and then says she feels dizzy and cannot stand up. She gives the mole as an excuse for not socialising. She says she thinks other girls see her as ugly and do not want to have anything to do with her. Recently she has even stopped wanting to see her only friend. Her mother is worried that Amrita will get a bad reputation. She and her husband will be looking for a husband for Amrita soon and she does not want the news to get around that her daughter has problems mixing.

### 7.6.1 Information about children who are excessively shy

These problems can show themselves in a number of different ways.

- Excessively shy children experience a fear of being looked at or of being ridiculed, embarrassed or humiliated.

- Some children are fearful of all social situations outside the home; others are just shy of particular social situations such as going to the temple or mosque.
- Most children with this problem will have been shy from a very early age. They may well be 'temperamentally' shy or have inherited a tendency to be shy.
- Most children who are excessively shy would like to be more sociable. Children with the social problems linked to language difficulties in ASD (see p. 26) do not mind not having any friends. These children need to be assessed and treated differently.
- The problem of excessive shyness may show itself when a child first goes to school. Some 5- or 6-year-olds will not say a word in school for the first few weeks or months, although they may chatter away at home. These children are selectively mute. Nearly always they begin talking at school, at least in a limited way, by the end of their first year in school.
- The problem of shyness may surface again in adolescence when in many, but not all, communities young people are expected to broaden their horizons and socialise in a much greater variety of settings.

Shyness is only likely to be a significant problem in communities where children and adolescents are allowed to mix freely with others of their own age. In communities in which they live a very sheltered life and are expected to remain at home when they are not at school, shyness is not likely to be a problem.

## 7.6.2 Finding out more about children who are excessively shy

- Obtain an account both from the parent and from the child about the nature of the problem and how long it has lasted.
- Try to find out the circumstances in which the shyness shows itself.
- What makes the shyness better or worse?
- To what degree is it interfering with the child leading a normal life?
- How would the child think life would be changed if he was less shy?
- See whether the child really wants to change, or whether he is happy with the way things are.

Now, given the information you have obtained, try to understand how the unusual degree of shyness has arisen in this particular child. Then go on to work out a plan to help.

## 7.6.3 Helping children who are excessively shy

If the child does not really want to change, then the health professional's ability to help is likely to be limited. Her most useful role may be to help the mother come to terms with the fact that she has a shy child who can nevertheless lead a reasonably normal life. The child may have a version of ASD (see Section 4.6).

If, however, the child wishes to receive some advice on how to overcome shyness, then try desensitisation. This involves helping children or adolescents to gradually overcome their fears, little by little. Help the child to first cope with the social situations he finds least upsetting. Then gradually move towards more and more stressful situations. For example, the following desensitisation programme might be suitable for a 14-year-old living in a Westernised community when he is given freedom to visit the homes of his friends:

- going with a friend to another friend's house to listen to some music – do this two or three times
- going without a friend to another friend's house to do the same
- going out to a café with two or three friends – do this two or three times

- going to a friend's house where there are six or seven friends having a party
- going to a stranger's house where there are some friends but also quite a lot of people he has not met before.

Another technique that can be used is imagining the worst situation. The child or adolescent could be asked to imagine what would happen if he went to a friend's house and the worst possible thing happened to him. What would that be? For example, would it be that no one would talk to him or that he might overhear someone say he was ugly or 'stuck-up'? What would he do in those circumstances? Could he work out how he could start a conversation with someone he had not met before by saying 'I don't know many people here, do you?', or 'How do you know (the host)?' or 'How do you feel about this sort of music? What is your favourite sort of music?'

If the child really does have, for example, a facial disfigurement, then one would need to help him develop a somewhat different set of skills. The child could ask a friend to introduce him to some strangers, who have been told about him beforehand. Maybe she would then be seen as a person who attends school X, has a favourite pop group, etc., instead of a boy with a facial disfigurement.

In motivated children these simple techniques may be very helpful.

Now make a list of the ways in which the health professional might be able to help Amrita.

## 7.7 Depression, misery and unhappiness

### Case 7.6
Benazir is a 14-year-old girl brought to a health clinic in the city by her mother because she is having headaches. It turns out the headaches are not much of a problem. But her mother says that for the past 6 months Benazir has been very moody and unhappy. This is not like her at all. Normally she is a bubbly girl with lots of friends who loves playing with her 4-year-old brother. Now she does not want to see her friends and shows no interest in her brother. She often tries to get out of going to school by saying she has a headache. She refuses to go to the mosque. She gets angry and irritable very easily. Her mother thinks that maybe she is being bullied at school or that she has lost her friends there. Maybe they are picking on her. Her schoolwork remains good. Nothing the mother can think of has upset her at home. What should the health professional do?

### Case 7.7
Leo is an 8-year-old boy who was brought to a health professional with stomach pains. But his mother said to the health professional that these were not at all serious and that the real problem was his difficult and disobedient behaviour for the past year. He gets extremely angry if he cannot get his own way. He sometimes cries for no good reason and will not go out to play with his friends when they come to call. This all started shortly after a set of losses that clearly upset him. His father went to another town some distance away to get work and only comes home about once every 3 months. His grandmother, of whom he was fond and who lived with the family, became ill and suddenly died. Before these unhappy events he was not at all a difficult boy. When the health professional first spoke to him he seemed quite happy talking about what he liked doing in school, but when she asked 'Tell me about your father' he immediately began to cry and said how much he missed him.

## 7.7.1 Information about depression, misery and unhappiness

Short periods of misery and unhappiness are common throughout childhood and adolescence. When such feelings are prolonged and intense it is appropriate to think of clinical depression. There is no sharp dividing line between ordinary misery and unhappiness and clinical depression.

Children show clinical depression in many different ways, partly depending on their age. As children get older they are better able to describe their moods and what is upsetting them. But even very young children have clinical depression, even if they cannot describe it themselves. They may show their depression by their appearance and behaviour. Definite signs of clinical depression are:

- feeling miserable, unhappy or sad
- lack of energy
- not wanting to do things that are normally enjoyed, such as seeing friends
- saying life is not worth living or wishing to be dead
- making a suicidal attempt.

Indicators to possible clinical depression (but may be normal or signs of other problems) include:

- losing appetite
- poor sleep
- boredom
- tiredness
- unexplained physical symptoms such as headache or stomach ache
- irritability and being easily roused to anger
- reluctance to go to school
- quality of schoolwork deteriorating
- drinking alcohol or taking drugs
- running away from home.

## 7.7.2 Causes of depression

These include physical causes (e.g. chronic infection, malnutrition, anaemia, viral illnesses, hormonal problems such as low levels of thyroid hormones) and losses (e.g. death of a loved family member or close friend, separation from a loved family member or close friend, loss of a pet, loss of self-esteem or confidence because of failure at school, or some other disappointment). Some children become depressed more easily than others. This may be because they have:

- a strong inherited genetic tendency to depression
- a sensitive temperament and are easily 'put out'
- suffered losses earlier in their lives.

Some children are resilient and do not get depressed even after multiple setbacks.

## 7.7.3 Finding out more about children who might be depressed

Mothers bringing children who are depressed to a health professional are unlikely to say that they think their child is depressed. They may not have noticed the signs or they may be too guilty or embarrassed to mention it. It is up to you to ask the right questions and to observe the child to see whether there are any signs of clinical depression. Probe further if:

- a child looks miserable or unhappy
- there is no physical cause for the problem with which the child has presented.

Good questions to ask mothers if you think a child may be depressed are:

- 'Do you think X has been low or "under the weather" recently?'
- 'Has X still been wanting to do things he usually enjoys?'
- 'Have you had the idea that X really feels life is not worth living?'

Children who might be clinically depressed should, if possible, be seen separately from their parents. Good questions to ask children over the age of 7 or 8 years (after setting them at ease by talking about neutral topics) might include:

- 'What sort of things do you like doing with your friends? Do you still enjoy those things?'
- 'What is it you've been most upset about recently?' NOT 'Have you been upset about anything recently?', as this allows them to avoid talking about painful subjects.
- 'Do you sometimes think that people don't like you very much? What makes you think that?'
- 'Do you feel you've done something bad?' and 'What might that be?'
- 'How do you feel about the future?' and 'Do you feel hopeless about what is going to happen to you?'

This may lead to questions probing suicidal thoughts and actions (see Section 9.4 on self-harm for suggested further questions).

Note that most children who are depressed also often show severe anxiety. Some may also show antisocial behaviour.

Now, given the information you have obtained, try to understand how unhappiness, misery and depression has arisen in this particular child. Then go on to work out a plan to help.

## 7.7.4 Helping children who may be depressed

In deciding whether to intervene in children who are depressed, you need to ask yourself these questions:

- Is the child's life being affected by their sadness, misery or depression?
- Does the child's thinking reveal guilt about the past, unrealistic ideas about not being liked or being worthless, or hopelessness about the future?
- Is there any risk of the child harming himself?

If the child is unhappy but low mood is not affecting his life – he can still go to school, participate in lessons, play with his friends and cope at home – and if, in addition, there is no evidence of distorted thinking, then there is no need for any active treatment. This does not mean you should not take his problems seriously. In particular, you should give him the opportunity to talk about what is upsetting him and try to reduce any stresses affecting him, as well as continue to monitor him.

If depression is affecting the life of the child but he is not, as far as you can see from the answers to the above questions, in any danger of harming himself, then you should try to work out what is upsetting him. In doing this you should always work in partnership with the child and parents. Can you help, for example, to:

- put a stop to any bullying
- reduce stress caused by schoolwork or examinations
- help parents to argue less

- help parents with their own mental health problems such as depression or anxiety
- reduce alcohol consumption in one or both of the parents.

Remember that depression following a loss does gradually improve as time goes on. A loss may make a child (or indeed any of us) feel that life will never be the same again after such a dreadful thing has happened. Yet we know that usually within a few weeks or months, deep, unhappy feelings will nearly always have reduced. This does not mean that a child is exactly the same person as beforehand. Losses do affect us, so a child may become better able to cope with loss when it happens again or, in contrast, more vulnerable to depression.

As well as reducing stress there are special forms of listening and talking treatments that can help to shorten the episodes. If there is a psychologist available to provide CBT, a referral should be made. If there is no such help, the health professional may benefit from knowing the principles of CBT:

- develop a positive relationship with the child
- explain that sometimes depressed feelings come about because of negative or unrealistic thinking
- discuss any ideas of guilt, worthlessness and feelings of not being liked
- discuss the evidence that the child is using to confirm these distorted thoughts
- ask the child to keep a record of when these thoughts occur, in what circumstances they arise and what he does about them
- look at the record the child has kept and discuss whether it does really confirm or refute the thoughts he is experiencing.

In many cases this approach will result in the child realising that the thoughts experienced are unrealistic. This may be followed by a lifting of mood.

Note that sometimes depressive feelings and thoughts come apparently without cause or following an illness, especially a viral infection. Post-viral depression is not uncommon and can be very severe. Suspect this if the child was normal before the depression, there is a history of a viral illness, and no stresses have occurred that are severe enough to account for the depressive feelings.

---

**Case 7.8**

Abhik is a 14-year-old boy brought to the health professional by his mother because he is completely lacking in energy and unable to go to school. He was fine and doing well in school until about 2 months ago when he developed a temperature, aches and pains in his limbs, and feelings of exhaustion. He did not have any treatment and gradually the temperature went down and the aches and pains disappeared. However, he remained extremely tired and lethargic, did not want to eat, felt miserable and unhappy, and just wanted to lie in bed all day. He has been in this state for about 6 weeks and the health professional was unable to find any physical illness. He no longer had a temperature.

---

In cases where attempts at stress reduction and a psychological approach are ineffective or do not appear appropriate because of the absence of relevant stresses, the use of antidepressant medication, if it is available, should be considered (see Appendix 2).

For children who have suicidal thoughts or who are actively suicidal, further information is provided in Section 9.4.

# 7.8 Obsessions and compulsions

**Case 7.9**

Amr is a 13-year-old boy brought to the clinic by his very anxious mother. For the past year or so, according to his mother, Amr has been developing a number of funny habits. The worst is that he will not sit down in a chair at home. To begin with it was just one chair he would not sit in, but now he will not sit in any chair. He has also become extremely preoccupied with cleanliness, spending ages in the bathroom, especially after he has been to the toilet. In the morning he seems to need an hour in the bathroom. This is a Hindu household and each of the family members worship in front of the household deity for about 10 minutes a day. Amr kneels in front of the image, chanting mantras for longer and longer periods, in the evening for up to an hour. He also takes ages to get to bed, needing to check that his sheet is clean and all his clothes are in exactly the right place before he is happy to settle to sleep. Things seem to be getting worse, with longer and longer periods of praying and checking everything is in order before he will do anything at all. What should the health professional do?

## 7.8.1 Information about obsessions and compulsions

Obsessions are ideas that keep coming into the mind and will not go away even when you try to stop thinking about them. Compulsions are behaviours one has to repeat over and over again despite trying to stop, usually because of an idea that something bad will happen if one does not do them. It is normal for young children to show rituals or do things in a particular way. For example, children may avoid the cracks along the pavement or may need to line up their possessions in a special way. These types of behaviour are only a problem if they take a great deal of time and prevent the child from living a normal life. Children who have a problem of this type commonly have a fear of germs, which drives them to wash their hands repeatedly, over and over again, until the skin of their hands becomes dry and cracked.

Affected children often involve their parents or other people in their rituals. For example, they may constantly ask their parents for reassurance that they are clean and not contaminated by germs. They might have a recurring worry that their parents are going to die and repeatedly ask their parents if they are feeling well. They may show compulsive religious observance, praying for much longer periods than is usual in their community.

The problem may start in children as young as 6, but usually starts later in childhood or adolescence and occasionally may begin after an unpleasant or stressful experience.

Other members of the family, especially a parent, may have the problem and there may be a strong genetic influence. Adults who have this problem experience a great deal of inner resistance. One part of their mind struggles to stop the obsession or compulsion but another will not allow this to happen. Children seem to show less inner resistance than adults.

Children with these problems may also have tics (rapid repeated movements of the face or body such as eye-blinking – see Section 6.6). They are quite likely to be shy, inhibited children and very likely to be anxious and may also be depressed.

Children and adolescents who have this problem often deny that it exists, even though it is obviously affecting their lives. If the child and parents are keen for help, appropriate treatment can often be very effective. Without treatment these problems come and go, but can last for years and seriously affect the child's life.

## 7.8.2 Finding out more about children with obsessions/compulsions

- Find out when the problems began, whether anything seemed to trigger them off, how often they occur now, how they affect the child's life, and what seems to make them better or worse.

- Check for other problems such as tics, anxiety or depression, which are often present as well.
- It is important to try to see and talk to the child separately from the parents, but remember that the child may deny such problems even though they are seriously affecting his life.
- Find out to what degree the lives of other members of the family are affected by the child's problems. In order to carry out his compulsive behaviours the child may have succeeded in manipulating other members of the family to change quite considerably what they normally do.
- Find out how much the child wants to change the obsessions and/or compulsions that are affecting his life. There may be surprisingly little desire to change.

Now, given the information you have obtained, try to understand how obsessions and compulsions have arisen in this particular child. Then go on to work out a plan to help.

## 7.8.3 Helping children with obsessions/compulsions

Before any specific form of treatment is started, health professionals should try to help children to talk about their fears. They should explain that such fears are quite common and often occur because children are frightened of losing control of what happens to them. They are not a sign of madness. As they gain control of their behaviour, so they will become less frightened. There are three approaches to helping:

1 behavioural methods
2 medication
3 a combination of behavioural methods and medication. This is the most effective approach, but if, for some reason, only one of these is available, a reasonably good outcome can be achieved.

Both behavioural methods and medication are best carried out in specialist centres, but if such centres are not available, as will usually be the case, the health professional is likely to be able to help at least to some extent.

The most effective behavioural approach is known as response prevention. This can be carried out in two steps.

1 Exposure to the feared situation. For example, the child frightened of contamination by germs may be exposed to soil or dirty dishes, first just by looking at them and then by holding or touching them for longer and longer periods of time. The parents or health professional can model this behaviour, doing it herself and showing the child that no harm follows.
2 Prevention of the ritual. This might involve parents and others encouraging the child not to carry out her rituals for longer and longer periods of time. Gradually, the child will be able to control herself and will not need encouragement from others.

Regarding medication, useful agents include a selective serotonin reuptake inhibitor such as fluoxetine, starting with 20 mg (maximum dose of 80 mg in an older adolescent), or a tricyclic antidepressant such as clomipramine, at a dose of 3 mg/kg, up to a maximum of 100 mg in two divided doses (see Appendix 2 for a list of medications). There may also be a need for the treatment of tics, anxiety and/or depression (see Sections 6.6, 7.3 and 7.7).

Both children and parents should be encouraged to continue to talk about their fears as to what will happen if the obsessions or compulsive behaviour stops.

Now make a list of the ways in which the health professional might be able to help Amr.

CHAPTER 8

# Behaviour and related problems

Behaviour problems include:

- physically aggressive behaviour such as bullying, constantly getting into fights and hitting other people for no good reason
- disobedience and temper tantrums
- non-physical aggression such as teasing, name-calling and humiliating other people
- lying to cover up behaviour for which the child is worried he may get into trouble or for some other reason
- stealing from home, school or in the neighbourhood; it may be carried out in isolation or with other young people
- fire-setting that can be very minor or extremely destructive
- truancy, not because of anxiety but because the child really does not like school and thinks he can do more things he enjoys outside of school.

## 8.1 Temper tantrums and disobedience

### 8.1.1 Information about temper tantrums and disobedience

A temper tantrum is an outburst, usually occurring when a young child is frustrated and cannot get what he wants. It involves shouting, screaming and sometimes aggressive behaviour towards the person who is not giving the child what he wants. It can last anything from a minute or two to an hour. Sometimes the tantrum progresses to a breath-holding attack. In the worst of these, a child may actually go blue from lack of air.

Most children under the age of 5 or 6 years have an occasional temper outburst and this is quite normal. Children who have frequent temper outbursts (several a day) are often very disobedient and aggressive. Disobedient children may also be unusually active with difficulties in concentration (see Section 8.2). Young disobedient children with frequent temper tantrums are often also anxious, not liking to be left with strangers and generally easily upset.

There are usually several reasons why young children are disobedient and have frequent temper tantrums.

- The core of the problem usually lies in inconsistent parental control of a young child who is temperamentally 'difficult'.
- The mother may find it difficult to be firm and consistent because she is depressed and/ or has an impulsive personality.
- The parental relationship may be unhappy, so that the parents cannot agree on how to handle the problem.

- Parents may react to the child's problems by becoming impatient, aggressive and/or rejecting, or these attitudes may have been there from the start.

Discipline may be difficult to enforce because the family is living in overcrowded circumstances. There may be nowhere for the child to play, with worries about disturbing the neighbours.

Some severely disobedient children go on to develop severe aggressive behaviour in middle childhood and adolescence. On the other hand, others whose parents get 'on top' of the problem, calm down and show no unusual difficulties later on.

**Case 8.1**

Rishi was brought by his mother to the clinic at the age of 4.5 years because of frequent temper outbursts. She said that he had always been a 'difficult' child and seemed more irritable than other babies even shortly after his birth. But over the past year things have become worse. She cannot take him anywhere because if he cannot get what he wants, he often shouts, screams and tries to hit her. She usually gives in to him and then eventually he calms down. She has tried smacking him really hard but that does not seem to work – he just carries on screaming. All this happens several times a day. She feels so guilty and ashamed in the village store when he has an outburst because she feels everyone is looking at her, thinking what a terrible mother she is. As well as the tantrums he is generally disobedient and naughty. He is aggressive to his 2-year-old brother, hitting him at every opportunity when his mother is not looking. He makes a fuss at meals and will not go to bed when he is told to. His concentration is poor, although he seems to be quite a bright child. The mother said she felt like she is at the end of her tether. Her husband is a quiet, gentle man who is always giving in to Rishi. Her mother-in-law is very critical of her, saying she is not bringing up Rishi properly. She did not have this sort of problem with her children. What should the health professional do?

## 8.1.2 Finding out more about disobedient children with temper tantrums

- Obtain a clear account of the nature of the problem. Find out how often the temper tantrums occur, what brings them on, how long they last, what actually happens during the outbursts, how they are brought to an end and what happens afterwards.
- Do the same type of history-taking for disobedient behaviour, which is often present as well.
- What, if any, other problems are there: aggressive behaviour; hyperactivity and short attention span; anxiety at separation?
- What have the parents done about the problems so far? How do they behave when the child is clearly building up to a tantrum?
- How do the parents get on? Can they agree on how to handle the tantrums and disobedience?

- Are there any mental or physical health problems in the family? In particular, is the mother depressed?
- What is the child's level of development (see Section 4.1)? In particular, is there a delay in speech? If the child is going to school, are there any problems at school? Do the teachers see his behaviour as a problem?
- What are the home circumstances? Is the family pressed financially?

Now, given the information you have obtained, try to understand why this particular child has temper tantrums and is so disobedient. Then go on to work out a plan to help.

### 8.1.3 Helping a disobedient child with temper tantrums

Check which of the behaviour problems the parents would like to tackle first and possible barriers to successful intervention – for example, parents unlikely to agree together, the mother is too depressed to cooperate. If these are present, try to tackle these first (see Sections 1.4 and 14.1 on depression in parents and marriage problems respectively).

If possible, ask the mother to describe exactly how the behaviour problems start. What triggers them? Usually this will be the child not getting his own way. Can the mother tell when the child is 'building up' to a tantrum? What does she do when the child refuses to do what he is told or is about to have a tantrum? Has she tried distracting the child by giving him something to do that will take his mind off what he wants to happen? Does she reward the child when he is disobedient or has a tantrum by eventually giving in and letting him have his way? Suggest that the parents follow the rules below.

- Always try to avoid situations that bring about disobedience or tantrums by diverting the child's attention.
- If the child is clearly going to have a tantrum because diversion has not worked, then try to remove the child from the situation as soon as possible by, for example, taking him out of the village store.
- Talk to the child calmly and explain that, no matter how long his tantrum lasts, he is not going to get what he wants.
- When the tantrum is over, explain to the child that when he has another one he still will not get what he wants.
- Remember to reward the child for good behaviour, for example for not having a temper tantrum for a whole half-day. A star chart (Appendix 1) can be used for doing this.
- Tackle other problems such as disobedience at meals in a similar way.

Suggest that the parents try to build into the day some 'quality time', perhaps half an hour, which they will spend entirely with their child, doing things he really wants to do. Using this approach, it is likely that the problems will improve, although the child may well remain more difficult than most.

Now make a list of the ways in which the health professional might be able to help Rishi.

## 8.2 Hyperactivity and attention problems (ADHD)

### Case 8.2

Atif is 8 years old. His mother brought him to the clinic at the request of his teacher, who thought he might have some brain damage. The teacher told his mother that they have never had such a hyperactive boy in the school. He just cannot sit still or concentrate on anything. This was affecting his learning, which was falling behind. His mother, who was a cheerful, tolerant, rather restless woman herself, said she did not find him too much of a problem. He was indeed very active and always had been from a baby. She just let him play in the street to let off steam if he could not settle in the home. He could not concentrate on books for more than a moment or two, but neither could her husband who had also been hyperactive when he was a boy. Atif was at an average level in his school subjects but did not have many friends as he was always interfering in what other children were doing. While he was being talked about, Atif was quite well behaved, but when the health professional gave him some paper and coloured pencils, he was only able to concentrate on drawing for a few seconds.

### Case 8.3

Mohammed's mother brought her 7-year-old son to the clinic because she thought he had ADHD, which she had read about in the newspaper. She thought there might be a tablet to cut down his hyperactivity. He wanted to be outside playing football all the time. He did not seem able to concentrate on looking at a book for more than 15 minutes. His older sister had been able to read a book for an hour at his age. The school did not think there was a problem but the mother thought that maybe the school was covering things up. The health professional noticed that while she was talking to his mother, Mohammed was quite happy, sitting quietly looking at a magazine she had in the room.

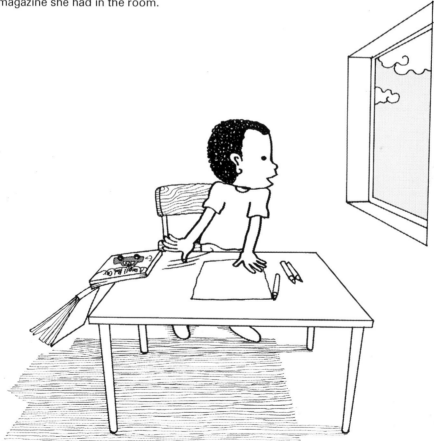

Although Atif clearly had a problem that required attention, Mohammed was just an active boy whose mother needed help to realise that her child's pattern of behaviour was quite normal for a boy of his age.

## 8.2.1 Information about hyperactivity and attention problems

Normal children vary widely in their level of activity and attention span. Genes play a major part in how active children are. However, children of parents who are not very good at setting limits are likely to be more active, especially if they have inherited 'overactive' genes. Often, though, the child's behaviour is a result of an interaction between genetic influences and one or more of the factors mentioned below, and as the child gets older, aggressive antisocial behaviour may begin to show itself. Generally, boys are affected three or four times as often as girls.

Children who are hyperactive will show a number of the following problems.

- The child will sometimes have been a restless infant, showing difficulties with feeding and sleeping. Speech and language delay may also be present.
- Inability to sit still for more than a few moments even in situations like school where children are expected to sit quietly for longer periods.
- A short attention span which means that they cannot concentrate on any task that requires some effort for more than a minute or two. They can, however, often sit still in front of a television for a longer period of time, especially if the programme is fast-moving, as this is such a passive activity requiring no effort. Many children can stay focused on a task for longer periods of time if it is their favourite activity, for example a computer game.
- Distractibility. The child's attention is easily distracted so that he cannot keep his mind on one thing at a time.
- Impulsive. The child behaves without thinking. Combined with clumsiness, this may mean the child is accident-prone.

Causes of hyperactivity/attention problems include:

- genetic factors: these are particularly strong in this condition
- brain dysfunction: children with epilepsy and cerebral palsy are especially likely to show hyperactivity
- prematurity and low birth weight
- chemical abnormalities in the brain
- poor social conditions with poverty and overcrowding
- unsettled early childhood experiences
- parents who are unresponsive to their child's demands
- diet: some children respond badly to sweet fizzy drinks as well as food additives such as colourings and preservatives
- other physical conditions such as ear problems, including recurrent infections or middle-ear effusion (see Section 12.3) and obstructive sleep apnoea (see p. 43), may also be relevant.

## 8.2.2 Finding out more about children with hyperactivity/attention problems

- There is no blood or urine test for ADHD. Even if investigations of brain function are available (and in most places they are not), these will not help in deciding whether the child is showing abnormal behaviour. Instead, you have to rely on the account given by the parents and teachers and on your own observations.
- Ask the parent questions about how long the child can concentrate on looking at a book, sit at the table for a meal, remain involved in a sitting-down activity that really interests him.
- Find out from the teachers how well the child is able to concentrate at school, compared with other children of the same age.

- Observe yourself how well the child can concentrate when you give him a task. The task might be to draw a picture or do a jigsaw appropriate for his age. Note, though, that some children with ADHD can focus remarkably well on the first visit.
- Especially where the problems are predominantly of poor attention, consider or check whether the child has hearing problems (see Section 12.3), iron deficiency, or behaviours suggesting the underlying problem may be more due to ASD (see Section 4.6), underlying specific developmental delay (see Chapter 4) or intellectual disability (see Chapter 5)
- Is the child reported to be clumsy? This may be due to poor attention or impulsiveness but some children with underlying coordination difficulties can cause concern because of their fidgetiness and poor behaviour (see Section 4.5)
- Has the child got other symptoms such as tics (see Section 6.6) or does he show antisocial behaviour (see Section 8.3 on aggressive behaviour and conduct disorder)? You then need to decide whether the child really does have a problem with attention and concentration.

Now, given the information you have obtained, try to understand how the overactivity and attention problems have arisen in this particular child. Then go on to work out a plan to help.

## 8.2.3 Ways of helping children with attention problems

Some parents, like Mohammed's mother (Case 8.3), think their children have an abnormal level of activity when their behaviour is well within the normal range. They have a mistaken view of normal activity levels. In these cases the mother needs reassurance but no further action is needed.

When the child's behaviour interferes with learning at school or is leading to the child being unable to sit still or to concentrate on a book, puzzle or drawing at home for more than a minute or two, there is a need to intervene, but always remember to ask what the parents have already tried.

Various simple measures should be suggested. First, explain about normal levels of activity and how this child falls outside those limits. The child will probably always show high levels of activity but it will be possible to make an improvement. Second, parents may be advised to:

- try to keep to a regular routine with the child, always doing things in the same order;
- tell the child about any changes of plan beforehand;
- give praise when there is any improvement in the child's behaviour;
- avoid punishment – the child is not to blame for being overactive;
- keep things simple: only make one request at a time so that the child does not have to keep too many things in his mind at once. Follow up on instructions, ensuring that the child complies with the request or instruction. Praise and or reward compliance;
- avoid overstimulation: play with one friend at a time, take part in one activity at a time. Avoid background television and radio. Do not go to crowded places such as markets or the village store at a busy time unless this is unavoidable;
- allow plenty of outdoor play in the street or fields to 'blow off steam';
- avoid fizzy drinks and foods with additives (e.g. heavily coloured sweets, fish fingers) if they seem to make things worse.

Third, suggest to teachers that they:

- give praise and reward even for small improvements in the child's ability to sit still and concentrate
- avoid punishment or humiliating the child – it is not the child's fault he is hyperactive
- give him one thing to do at a time

- make sure tasks given to the child are short, and if he stays on a task for more than a brief period, that he is praised
- make sure your instructions are simple and clear
- sit the child in the front of the class so that you can keep an eye on him
- make sure he is sitting next to 'good' children who will not encourage him to get into trouble.

If the child's behaviour is still causing significant problems, then, if it is available locally, a trial of medication may be helpful. The drugs usually given are methylphenidate or atomoxetine (see Appendix 2). However, these drugs have a number of side-effects and should only be prescribed by a specialist children's doctor.

Star charts (Appendix 1) can be used both at home and at school to reward desirable behaviours. The child may be encouraged to stay focused on a specific activity for gradually increasing periods of time, and rewarded for doing so. If, with your help, parents and teachers can help to keep the child from being discouraged and angry because he feels nobody likes him, the outcome may be good.

Hyperactive children who develop antisocial behaviour because they have been unsympathetically treated or have drifted towards other children who have a bad influence on them will often have serious problems later on.

Now make a list of the ways in which the health professional might be able to help Atif and Mohammed.

## 8.3 Aggressive behaviour and bullying

**Case 8.4**

Ajit is a 10-year-old boy brought to the clinic by his mother because the school has complained about his behaviour and has told the mother she must take him to the clinic or he will not be allowed in school again. Yesterday he really hurt another boy, whose mother complained about him and said something must be done. Ajit always seems to be in a fight. His mother says that he complains about other boys picking on him and that he never starts a fight, but the teachers say this is not true. He has an older brother who has also been in trouble for fighting. Ajit is behind in his schoolwork compared with the other children in his class because he can hardly read. His father is a labourer who is in regular work, but he drinks heavily and when he comes home at night he is sometimes violent. Ajit is frightened of him. His father beats him with a stick when he is in trouble at school but it does not seem to make any difference. What should the health professional do?

### 8.3.1 Information about aggressive behaviour and bullying

Aggressive behaviour takes two main forms.

1 Physical force against other people, especially other children. Fighting is the use of force against others of the same size; hitting smaller children is bullying.
2 Hurtful teasing and humiliation of other people, especially other children. Calling names and spreading malicious stories are two common ways in which this occurs. Such behaviour may be face to face or behind the victim's back. Nowadays, it may take the form of cyberbullying on the internet or by texting on mobile telephones.

Being a victim of bullying at school is a major source of stress for a significant number of schoolchildren.

Aggressive behaviour may occur at home, within the family, at school or in the neighbourhood. Physical aggression is more commonly shown by boys; teasing and humiliation more by girls. Fighting and bullying may be undertaken alone or in groups or by neighbourhood gangs. There are two main types of aggressive behaviour shown by individual children:

1   impulsive, i.e. triggered by a perceived attack
2   controlled, i.e. planned.

Children who show impulsive physical aggression often have problems with attention, concentration and learning (see Section 8.2). Note also that children with aggressive behaviour may have quite deep depressive feelings and may show their aggression particularly when they are feeling low in mood. They may also show other forms of antisocial behaviour, such as truancy, stealing, lying and fire-setting. When these behaviours occur together, it is called conduct disorder.

There may be feelings of inferiority arising, for example, from being small in height, having a chronic physical problem or being a slow learner.

Impulsive, aggressive behaviour often begins in the early years but frequently persists into later childhood and adolescence, and occasionally into adulthood. The background features of children with aggressive behaviour include:

* difficult, overactive behaviour in infancy and early childhood
* models of aggressive behaviour in the home, especially fathers and older brothers
* being members of large families, living in overcrowded conditions
* the frequent use of physical force rather than reasoning as a form of discipline at home
* discipline at home that is inconsistently enforced
* learning difficulties
* attendance at schools at which fighting between children commonly occurs and is even tolerated
* exposure to violent images in the media.

Most children who show aggressive behaviour do not have evidence of brain damage, but children with epilepsy and other evidence of brain dysfunction do have higher than expected rates of aggressive behaviour.

## 8.3.2 Finding out more about children with aggressive behaviour

* Some of this information is best obtained from the child seen alone. If it is possible to see the child before the parents, this may reduce the child's level of suspiciousness.
* Obtain an account of the aggressive behaviour to find out when it began, where it shows itself, how often it occurs, and how it is triggered.
* How serious is the behaviour? Has the child inflicted serious injury on anyone? Does he use a weapon?
* What does the child feel about his behaviour? Is he guilty or does he usually think his aggression has been justified by the way he has been treated by other children?
* What is the method of discipline in the home? Is beating a frequent form of punishment?
* Do the parents agree on the form of rewards and punishments that are used in the home?
* Does the child have any underlying depressive feelings? What seems to make him depressed? Does he have a poor self-image because of being small or having a physical illness or being behind at school?
* Does the child have any other antisocial behaviour such as truancy, stealing, fire-setting or problems with attention and concentration?
* How is the child getting on in his schoolwork?

- What is the school's attitude to aggressive behaviour? Is it tolerated or taken very seriously?
- Does the child watch a lot of violent television programmes or play computer games with violent themes?

Now, given the information you have obtained, try to understand how the aggressive behaviour has arisen in this particular child. Then go on to work out a plan to help.

### 8.3.4 Helping children with aggressive behaviour

Much of the responsibility for stopping bullying in schools lies with teachers and the school authorities (see Section 16.3 on anti-bullying programmes in schools). Dealing with aggressive behaviour more generally is also the responsibility of the school, the parents and the police (if it involves criminal activity or delinquency). A health professional with limited resources will be able to provide helpful input by bringing greater understanding to the problem, supporting the parents when they are behaving appropriately and identifying children in whom depressive feelings are an important reason why a child is being aggressive. It is unlikely that a health professional will be able to undertake interventions that significantly reduce most aggressive behaviour or bullying. However, useful interventions may include:

- counselling parents about the need for consistent discipline based on reward for good behaviour rather than punishment (see Chapter 15);
- seeing the child alone to discuss his attitude towards the trouble he is in, who he thinks is responsible, what he is going to do about it;
- seeing the child alone to check whether he has significant depressive feelings, and if so, how these may be increasing the likelihood of aggression;
- contacting the school to find out what their attitude is to fighting and bullying: offering advice on anti-bullying programmes (see Section 16.3);
- identifying whether there are any practical measures that can be taken to reduce feelings of inferiority, and to improve self-worth and self-confidence, such as extra help for reading or a club with facilities for vigorous activities such as football or boxing.

Now make a list of the ways in which the health professional might be able to help Ajit.

## 8.4 Fire-setting

### 8.4.1 Information about fire-setting

Setting fires is an unusual form of antisocial behaviour almost always involving boys. It may be carried out alone or with a group. If carried out with a group there is often a great deal of other antisocial behaviour such as breaking into property and fighting. Individual boys who set fires alone may do so because:

- they have a fascination with fire and matches, going back many years
- they feel a strong sense of anger because they think they have been rejected and want revenge
- they have delusions and hallucinations, with fire-setting arising as a result of psychotic symptomatology
- they are bored and crave excitement.

They often come from very disturbed homes that are disorganised and chaotic. There may be a history of psychosis in the family. Note that all children who play with fire need not have serious problems like Ahan (see below). However, they need to be supervised carefully and also be provided with distractions and opportunities to engage in other activities.

**Case 8.5**

Ahan is a 12-year-old boy brought along by the police, who have caught him setting a fire. They have brought him to the clinic because he has burnt one of his hands trying to avoid arrest and needs medical attention. There have been a number of fires in the district, some of which have caused a great deal of damage. The police have suspected Ahan because he has been seen near the scene of the other fires. They think that on one occasion he tried to set fire to his school building, but fortunately the smoke was spotted before any serious damage was done. This time they have caught him lighting a fire in a yard used for dumping rubbish. On one occasion the police tried to interview him at home and discovered that he lives with his mother, a very odd woman who talks to herself and seems to have visions. She is regarded as a witch by many of her neighbours. The school say that Ahan is an isolated boy and has no friends. After she has put a dressing on his hand, the health professional wonders whether there is more she can do.

## 8.4.2 Finding out more about a child who is thought to be fire-setting

If possible, the child should be seen alone as well as with his parents. Fire-setting may be part of a general pattern of antisocial behaviour carried out with other boys who are showing similar problems. If so, then proceed as with other types of antisocial behaviour such as aggression and stealing.

- Find out when the fire-setting began, how often it has happened, where it has occurred and what seems to trigger it.
- What is going through the boy's mind when he decides to start a fire?
- Does the boy have any signs of a psychotic illness (see Chapter 11)?
- What are the parents' attitudes to this behaviour? Do they show signs of mental illness?
- What is the quality of care in the home? Are there signs of neglect or other forms of abuse?
- How is the boy getting on in school? Information from his teachers about his educational progress and friendships or lack of them will be useful.

Now, given the information you have obtained, try to understand how the fire-setting and aggressive behaviour have arisen in this particular child. Then go on to work out a plan to help.

### 8.4.3 Helping children who have been responsible for fire-setting

If fire-setting is part of a general pattern of antisocial behaviour carried out with other boys who are showing similar problems, then proceed as with other types of antisocial behaviour such as aggression and stealing. Otherwise tailor the approach to the motivation shown by the boy. If the boy is showing signs of psychotic behaviour, then treat as per Chapter 11.

- If he is showing signs of rejection, then talk to his parents and the school about how he can be helped to make friends and engage in other activities. This is not likely to be easy as he may well show features of mild ASD (see Section 4.6) or intellectual disability.
- If the behaviour is repetitive and there seem to be triggers that set it off, then work out with the parents and the child as to how an alternative response can be developed.

Identify any stresses in the home, especially mental illness in parents, so that appropriate treatment can be provided. If the boy has feelings about his parents or other members of the family that he cannot communicate, try to work out ways in which he can be helped to express himself.

Fire-setting tends to be a repetitive form of behaviour and can cause a great deal of damage to property. If necessary (and it usually will be), try to arrange for the boy to be closely supervised in situations in which he has previously set fires.

Now make a list of the ways in which the health professional might be able to help Ahan.


## 8.5 Lying

### 8.5.1 Information about lying

There are various reasons why children and adolescents do not tell the truth. They may be:

- too young (under the age of 4 years) or not yet intelligent enough to know the difference between truth and untruth: note that children with intellectual disability, although of a chronologically higher age, may be functioning at a lower age level;
- spinning fantasies in imaginative play, for example a 4-year-old who says her doll really can talk may be unable to tell the difference between truth and fantasy;
- telling lies to cover something up, like Shreya (see p. 81);
- trying to impress other children by boasting, for example that their father owns a car when, in fact, he only owns a bicycle;
- getting out of trouble: for example when, after skipping school to play football with friends, a boy tells the teacher he has been sick in bed and may even forge a note he pretends has been written by his mother.

Possible underlying reasons for lying in older children who are capable of understanding the difference between truth and fiction include:

- parents who are involved in telling lies to each other or to those in authority, so that the child has poor role models
- an underlying sadness, as with Shreya
- lying being part of a widespread pattern of antisocial behaviour, including aggression, truanting and stealing
- fear of severe punishment if they are caught out in some form of disobedience or 'naughty' behaviour.

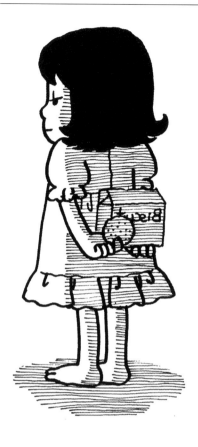

**Case 8.6**

Shreya is a 5-year-old girl brought to the health clinic by her mother, who had been told to bring her daughter by the teacher who thought something should be done about Shreya's weight. Shreya is now the weight of an average 9-year-old girl. But what is upsetting the mother is that Shreya is always telling lies. Her mother knows that Shreya constantly steals food. She even gets up at night to take food. Her mother has tried to put the food high up in places Shreya cannot reach. At about 1 o'clock in the morning the other night there was a thump and the mother walked into the kitchen to find that Shreya had fallen off a chair while trying to reach some food that her mother had put on a high shelf to stop her getting it. Shreya had hurt herself but even then denied that she had been on the chair trying to reach food. The health professional spent some time with the mother, trying to work out with her why Shreya had this compulsive need to eat. It started when her father left home about a year ago. Basically, Shreya is a very unhappy girl who eats to comfort herself. This is the real problem and the health professional tried to work out with the mother ways to deal with Shreya's sadness.

## 8.5.2 Finding out more about children who are lying

Lying is nearly always either a sign of immaturity or a symptom of some other problem. If the child is too young or immature to know the difference between fact and fiction, the parents can be reassured that as the child develops so the telling of lies will stop. They should, however, explain to the child the importance of telling the truth.

## 8.5.3 Helping children who are lying

If the lying is a symptom of some other problem, then it is important to try to tackle the underlying problem, such as misery, unhappiness or widespread antisocial behaviour. Guidance on helping children who have depression or antisocial behaviour is given in other sections.

Now make a list of the ways in which the health professional might be able to help Shreya.

# 8.6 Stealing

## 8.6.1 Information about stealing

The idea of personal property (what is mine is mine and what is yours is yours) does not really develop properly until the age of 5 years. Before this age when children take something that does not belong to them, they do not realise this is wrong and it cannot be regarded as stealing. All the same, when they do take something belonging to someone else it is important for parents to make clear that this is a wrong thing to do. There is no need for punishment; just a clear explanation.

Between 6 and 8 years, children may not have a very well-developed sense of property, so if they do take someone else's property, a telling off with an explanation is all that is required. After this age, a single episode of stealing can be seen just as a child seeing what he can get away with. But repeated stealing is a reason for concern.

Children of normal intelligence and over 8 years know that it is wrong to take other people's property, but they may not have sufficient control of their impulses to resist taking something they really want from another child or from home. Children may steal outside the home because they:

- are hungry and there is insufficient food at home to meet their needs
- have a sense of deprivation, perhaps because other children have prized possessions – new trainers, a mobile telephone, a games console – that they badly want for themselves
- are depressed and find it comforting to take something they really want from the cupboard at home, a shop or from another child
- comfort stealing – in cases of neglect, deprivation and lack of love, the child may engage in stealing as a way of compensating for deprivation or for psychological comfort
- crave attention – being noticed, even getting into trouble for stealing, may seem preferable to being ignored
- want to prove themselves as brave and risk-takers in front of other children.

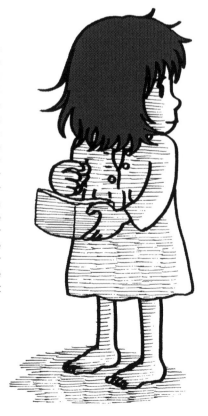

**Case 8.7**
Maya was a 10-year-old girl brought to the clinic because she had a skin infection, impetigo. She was clearly undernourished, small for her age and very miserable. What struck the health professional was that her mother was very angry with her. The health professional asked the mother why she was so angry. The mother replied that Maya kept on stealing money from her purse and she had done so only this morning. Maya was a very naughty girl; she knew her mother had very little money and yet she kept taking money that was meant for food. The health professional managed to see Maya by herself. She asked Maya what she did with the money she stole. Maya said she gave it to other girls in school. She had no friends, but if she gave money or little presents to the other girls they let her play with them. Maya had no pocket money like the other girls. She knew what she did was wrong but she could not stop herself.

Adolescents who steal in groups are likely to belong to delinquent gangs engaged in various forms of other antisocial activity, such as truancy (see pp. 84–86) and aggressive behaviour (see pp. 76–78). Adolescents who steal alone usually do so for the purpose of buying cigarettes, alcohol or illegal drugs. The child has acquired a drug habit that is too expensive for him to fund without stealing. If the drug intake has become addictive (see Section 10.2), then the stealing may involve quite large sums of money. Background features of children who steal include:

- material and/or emotional deprivation – lack of love and affection
- neglect with inadequate parental supervision
- other family members have been in trouble with the law
- educational retardation, especially difficulties in reading
- other antisocial behaviour, such as truancy and aggressive behaviour
- poor attention and concentration.

## 8.6.2 Finding out about a child who steals

The health professional will inevitably be seen by the child or teenager as an authority figure. This means that the child will see the health professional as someone who disapproves of him, and perhaps has the power to punish him or take him away from home. Consequently, it is especially important for the health professional to avoid making any judgements about the child's behaviour or to appear critical in any way. In order to reduce suspiciousness, it may be helpful to first see the child alone, before seeing a parent.

- Obtain some idea from the mother and child of the child's life at home and school. How does the child get on with any brothers and sisters? Does he have friends? What sort of things does he like to do? How is he getting on with schoolwork?
- Find out about the home circumstances – how many children are there, is there enough money to buy essentials?
- Assess the quality of care given to the child. Does he look clean or neglected compared with other children in the locality? Does the mother talk warmly about him or do you feel she thinks of him as a nuisance?
- Find out when the stealing began, where and how often it has occurred, what has been stolen, how any money that has been stolen has been used, how the parents or others have reacted?
- Are there any other behaviour or emotional problems? Is the child depressed? Alternatively, or perhaps in addition, the child may be showing other behaviour problems such as lying and fighting. School attendance needs checking as this may well be poor.
- Does he have problems with attention and concentration?
- What is the child's level of intelligence? Does he understand the difference between right and wrong?
- How does the child feel about having been caught stealing? Is he ashamed and guilty or rather proud of himself?
- What does the parent(s) think is the reason for the stealing? What action have they taken already?

Now, given the information you have obtained, try to understand why this particular child is stealing. Then go on to work out a plan to help.

### 8.6.3 Ways of helping children who steal

Dealing with stealing is the responsibility of the school, the parents and the police (if it involves criminal activity or delinquency). A health professional with limited resources will be able to provide helpful input by bringing greater understanding to the problem, supporting the parents in dealing with the problem appropriately, and identifying children in whom depressive feelings are an important reason as to why they are stealing.

The family may be in serious poverty, with the stealing arising from financial hardship. The health professional is not going to be able to inject more money into the home, but advice on household management or on how to spend the little money there is more effectively, may be helpful. Otherwise counsel the parents along the following lines (see also Chapter 15):

- It is important for them to give the child a clear message that stealing from other people is wrong and that they do not approve of it.
- Explain the possible consequences of continued stealing.
- If they are sure the child has stolen, do not ask the child to own up. This may just result in the child lying to cover up. Then the child has committed two offences instead of one.
- Can the child be given more attention, hugs and kisses? Is it possible for the mother or older brothers and sisters to spend more time with him?
- Can the parents try to make sure that any money in the home is made more secure so that it is not so easy to steal?
- The health professional might contact the school to see whether the child's teachers can do anything to help him make friends, to ensure he is included in games without having to buy friendship.
- Make sure the child is rewarded for good behaviour. Rewards need not be material; a hug and warm words may work better anyway.
- If it can be afforded, a small amount of regular pocket money will at least give the child the feeling that he has at least some money to spend as he likes.

Deal with any associated depressive feelings (see Section 7.7) or problems with attention and concentration (see Section 8.2).

If the stealing is seen as part of a widespread pattern of antisocial behaviour (including bullying, fighting, truancy and lying), usually undertaken with others, then this should be managed as described under Section 8.3.4.). It is very likely that the police will become involved at some point if the stealing has arisen to fund a drug habit (see Section 10.2).

If the child is slow to learn, contact the school to make sure the teachers are aware of any learning difficulties and are doing their best to help the child improve. Of course, many teachers will have too many children in their classes to give individual attention, but it may be possible for other children who are more advanced to give help if the child is accepting of this.

Now make a list of the ways in which the health professional might be able to help Maya.

## 8.7 Truancy

**Case 8.8**

Alaa is an 11-year-old boy brought by his mother to the clinic because he has fallen from a wall and hurt his ankle. He is limping quite badly but the health professional is able to rule out a fracture with an X-ray very quickly. While the health professional was bandaging the sprained ankle, she realised that the accident had happened at 11:00 on a mid-week morning when he should have been in school. She asked his mother why he had not been in school. His mother replied that she wished she knew. She suspected he had been skipping quite a lot of school. In fact, she had been to the school the previous week to ask about his progress and the teacher had said he was hardly ever in school. His mother had not known what to do about it and had told Alaa that he must go to school. But clearly Alaa had not obeyed her. There was no father in the home. An older brother had left school at 13 years and was working as a labourer's assistant, carrying bricks and making the tea. What should the health professional do?

## 8.7.1 Information about truancy

Truancy is frequent among boys who are in their last years of schooling and who do not find school a rewarding experience. It is different from school refusal. In truancy:

- parents do not know their children (usually boys) are missing school
- children are often in groups with other truants, involved in other forms of antisocial behaviour.
- children often have learning difficulties.

In contrast, children who are refusing to go to school:

- have difficulty separating from their parents
- are isolated and have few friends
- are anxious, often rather obsessional children
- do not cover up school absences from parents
- are usually intelligent and making good progress at school.

Background features of children who skip school (truants) include:

- educational retardation, especially backwardness in reading
- other antisocial behaviour, such as stealing, lying and aggressive behaviour
- poor attention and concentration
- neglect with inadequate parental supervision
- material and/or emotional deprivation – lack of love and affection
- other family members have been in trouble with the law.

Schools vary greatly in their attitude to children missing school for no good reason. Some do not have the resources to ensure unwilling children do attend; others have attendance officers who visit the home when a child is absent.

Children who skip school often find the curriculum unrewarding. Schools with few resources are unable to deliver the individual tuition necessary to ensure a child is receiving relevant education. Unless this can be provided, even if a successful attempt is made to get a truanting child back to school, the problem is likely to recur.

## 8.7.2 Finding out more about a child who is truanting

- As with other forms of antisocial behaviour, the child is likely to see the health professional as an authority figure who will be critical of him. If the health professional is to establish trust, she should not make judgements or be critical. If possible, it is a good idea to see the child first as this will reduce the child's level of suspiciousness.
- Find out when the child began to miss school. Was this related to any particular event, such as a change of teacher? What does the child do when out of school? What efforts has the school made to check on the child's attendance and get the child back to school? (Note that often the school will just not have the resources for this.)
- What is the child's educational level? Are there school subjects such as sport that he is good at?

- Does the child show attention and concentration problems (see Section 8.2)?
- What is the parents' attitude to the child missing school? Do they take it seriously or has their own experience perhaps led them to believe that school is a waste of time?
- What resources does the school have for dealing with children who are skipping school? The health professional's local knowledge will be very helpful here.

Now, given the information you have obtained, try to understand why this particular child is skipping school. Then go on to work out a plan to help.

## 8.7.3 Helping children who are truanting

Traunting is mainly a matter for the school and the school authorities. The health professional may, however, have a limited part to play.

- Treat any depression (see Section 7.7), anxiety (see Section 7.1), or attention and concentration problems (see Section 8.2).
- Inform the school of your concerns regarding school attendance.
- Be prepared to listen to parents who wish to talk about their child's problems.

Now make a list of the ways in which the health professional might be able to help Alaa.

# CHAPTER 9

# Specific problems in adolescence

## 9.1 Introduction

**Case 9.1**

Sixteen-year-old Abra's mother came to see a health professional saying she was worried about her son and that she could not sleep and was off her food. She said she could not concentrate on her office job; she was getting told off by her boss, who said she was making too many mistakes. She said that Abra had given up going to school, and did not have a job. He was smoking and drinking. She thought he was seeing a girl who was 'no good'. He always came home late at night and sometimes did not come home at night at all. She had no idea where he was. Then he would lie in bed in the morning saying he was too tired to get up. If she asked him to do some shopping, he snapped at her and told her he was not 'her slave'. His father gave him money, which was how he could afford the cigarettes and alcohol. She herself had attended a convent school with nuns as teachers and had been kept at home by strict parents in her teenage years and this was what she wanted to do with Abra, but it was impossible. She went to mass regularly, but Abra never came. Her husband said Abra was just a normal adolescent. Abra had never been very good at schoolwork and had often been in trouble at school, which he had left when he was 14. She felt the school had been quite pleased when Abra stopped attending. He had never been in trouble for breaking the law. What should the health professional do?

### 9.1.1 Information about adolescent problems

In most high-income countries, adolescence is defined as the period between puberty and adulthood, from about 13 to 19. In these countries it is often thought 'normal' for young people of this age to rebel against their parents and other authority figures and to become involved in risky behaviour such as drinking alcohol, smoking, taking drugs and engaging in sexual promiscuity. Other features thought to be normal in adolescence are irritability and mood swings. There are two relatively new features of normal adolescence seen in different countries and cultures.

1   Many young people, especially those in continuing education, are financially dependent on their parents not just during their teenage years, but into their mid-20s or even longer.
2   Spending of large amounts of time participating in various forms of social networking.

A child from a high-income country is more likely to experience adolescence as described above, as families are able to manage financially without their child's contribution. However, in families that depend on their children going to work at a young age (e.g. going to work in the fields), children may move from childhood to young adulthood without a phase of life in between.

A 'Western' type of adolescence is also absent in societies in which there are strong religious beliefs prohibiting the use of alcohol and early sexual experience. In such societies there is often a culture of early marriage, especially for girls, so that there is only a very short period between the onset of menstruation and marriage.

The physical changes of puberty occur during the teenage years (sometimes beginning even earlier). The behavioural and emotional changes often associated with adolescence vary greatly between societies. It is important for health professionals to be aware of the features of adolescence in the societies in which they work.

In most countries the rate of mental health problems is about the same in adolescence as it is in childhood and adult life. There are, however, some changes that begin to occur during this time.

- While before adolescence boys and girls experience emotional problems equally, during this period girls are more frequently affected.
- Certain serious mental illnesses such as schizophrenia and bipolar disorder (see Sections 11.1 and 11.2) are rare before adolescence but begin to occur more frequently during this time.
- Similarly, self-harm is unusual before adolescence but then begins to become more common.
- Where a Western type of adolescence exists, the roots of addiction to alcohol, tobacco and illicit drugs are often laid down at this time.

Because of the false idea that adolescence is necessarily a time of great emotional turbulence, some serious mental health problems may be regarded as normal and not considered significant. Teenagers who are disabled by emotional or behaviour problems are in just as great a need of attention to their mental health as in any other phase of life. It is sometimes said that teenagers resist the idea of attending healthcare clinics. Some certainly do, but the rate of adolescent attendance at health clinics is about the same as with older age groups.

As a result of the spread of Western culture, especially through the media, a Western type of adolescence as described earlier is now regarded as normal in many more parts of the world. This is particularly the case in urban areas in LAMI countries that are experiencing increasing prosperity.

Although the freedom, opportunities for exploration and enjoyment of the Western lifestyle of adolescence clearly have positive aspects, there are two major negative features.

1 Patterns of behaviour laid down during adolescence may be a major disadvantage later on. For example, it may be difficult later on for teenagers to accept the routine and self-discipline necessary to hold down a job in contemporary society.
2 The parents of teenagers who are living a rebellious, turbulent adolescence may themselves suffer mental health problems as a reaction.

### 9.1.2 Finding out about mental health problems in adolescence

The health professional needs to be aware of the various 'normal' ways in which teenagers behave in the society in which she is working. Note that in many societies where it is assumed that teenagers will be drinking or smoking heavily, on drugs, out of school, moody and rebellious to their parents, the majority may be leading lives nothing like this. They may be generally obedient and working hard at school, although they are very likely to be spending a considerable amount of time in social networking.

The same criteria should be used in deciding whether a young person has a mental health problem as at any other age. The first question to be asked is whether they are distressed or disabled in their daily lives by emotional and behaviour problems (see Section 3.1). The second question is what sort of problem do they have and how can they be helped. The approach should depend on the nature of the problem, as described in other sections of this book. 'Adolescent disorder' is not, in itself, a diagnosis.

Where a young person in their teenage years is showing a mental health problem, it is often difficult to encourage them to attend a clinic for assessment. In large cities there may be drop-in centres to which adolescents can refer themselves.

If young people do attend but are reluctant to say what is on their mind, it may be helpful just to get them to talk about their lives and how they see the future if they go on as they are. Most young people of this age prefer to be listened to and talked to as one would with an older adult. It is not a good idea to pretend to be familiar with teenage culture or to act as 'one of the boys/girls'.

When teenagers are living turbulent lives, it is often the parents who are suffering, with their adolescent children either quite happy with their lives or unwilling to ask for help. In these cases it may be the parents who attend a clinic, often with an emotional problem such as depression and/or anxiety. In exploring the reasons for their emotional state it becomes clear that a 'difficult' teenager is the focus of their concerns. Assessment of a mental health problem in a teenager may require finding out information from a parent who may, himself, need advice and counselling.

With younger adolescents it will always be a good idea to have a discussion with one of the child's teachers to find out how the young person is getting on at school.

### 9.1.3 Helping adolescents with mental health problems

If the young person is affected in everyday life by a mental health problem, the first challenge is to help him to accept that he does require help of some sort. The first step is to discuss with him what he feels is the matter and how he thinks he might be helped. This discussion will often make it clear what can be done. Often the young person feels that people other than himself are responsible for what is happening. The health professional can agree to discuss this issue to start with as an opportunity to negotiate for later follow-up visits.

Where the young person is not seeking help but one or both parents is seriously depressed or anxious about the matter, counselling should be provided for the parents.

Now make a list of the ways in which the health professional might be able to help Abra.

## 9.2 Sexual development

**Case 9.2**

Mandara is a 4-year-old girl brought to the clinic by her very anxious mother because she has caught Mandara playing a 'sex game' with a boy of the same age who lives next door. The two of them were half undressed, with their underwear off, in a field at the back of their dwellings looking at each other's genital areas when a passer-by saw them, brought them back to their homes and told their mothers very angrily what he had seen. Mandara's mother did not know what to do. There was nothing 'sexual' going on in the home. She and her husband were very careful not to walk about undressed in the home. She whispered to the health professional that when she and her husband 'had relations', which they hardly ever did, they always made sure the children were fast asleep. There were no other problems. What should the health professional do?

## 9.2.1 Information about sexual development

Sexual drive, the tendency to seek pleasure from stimulation of the genitalia, is present from birth, although there is a marked increase in this drive during adolescence. Before puberty, sexual drive varies greatly. It mainly shows itself by:

- sexual curiosity – boys and girls noticing the physical appearance of adults when naked and examining each other's genitalia
- masturbation or self-stimulation of the genitalia (penis and clitoris) to produce pleasurable sensations.

Both of these are normal activities.

Before puberty, children develop in their sexual thoughts and ideas in three main ways.

1  Gender identity. Thinking of oneself as boy or girl, male or female. By 2–3 years, most children have a strong sense of identity and this nearly always remains stable. A very small number of boys and girls have a gender identity which is the opposite of their anatomical gender: normal-looking girls have the fixed idea they are boys and vice versa.
2  Gender role behaviour. In most, but not all, societies, before puberty, boys and girls behave in different ways. For example, boys usually play with boys and girls with girls. Boys tend to be more physically adventurous and girls more interested in playing with dolls and in domestic activities. However, there are considerable differences between cultures in how important these differences are thought to be. It is not uncommon for girls to be tomboys and boys to be effeminate.
3  Sexual orientation. This refers to a child's preference for the same or opposite gender when achieving sexual arousal, especially in masturbation. By the beginning of adolescence sexual orientation is usually well established.

The first visible signs of puberty in girls (e.g. breast changes) usually occur between 8 and 13 years and a couple of years later in boys (e.g. pubic hair growth). In countries with poorer nutritional levels, these changes occur later, sometimes as much as 4 years later than stated. In general, pubertal changes from childhood to mature adulthood usually take around 5 years, but there is great variation both within societies and between societies in the ages at which puberty occurs.

Masturbation in adolescence is normal, although it is often condemned by adults. Many adolescents feel extremely guilty about masturbation because they have been brought up to believe it is harmful and wrong. It is, in fact, harmless.

The age when sexual behaviour between boys and girls or men and women normally occurs varies greatly between societies. Similarly, the frequency of sexual behaviour before marriage varies greatly: in some societies it is very common; in others it is very infrequent. In some societies where it is common, often girls in their early and mid-teens become pregnant, sometimes as a result of unprotected sexual intercourse, especially under the influence of alcohol. Pregnancy during adolescence has a number of marked disadvantages both for the young mother and for the baby: birth complications are more common, the mother may not be sufficiently mature to look after her child and her education may be irreversibly interrupted. Sexually transmitted diseases are relatively common in adolescents in some societies.

A small number of boys and girls discover during their early teenage years (or even earlier) that their sexual preference is for individuals of the same gender. Sometimes they do not have a marked sexual preference for one or other gender: they are bisexual. In both cases, sexual preference may change again during adolescence.

Often, young people will feel the need to keep their sexual orientation a secret if it does not conform to their family's or culture's beliefs. Young people with homosexual or bisexual preferences may come to the attention of health professionals because they are depressed or have even been involved in self-harming behaviour. Note that whatever the attitude to homosexuality in the society in which the health professional is working, he should not make moral judgements herself about whether such behaviour is right or wrong. She should provide whatever helps she can in an understanding way. Remember there are no interventions that can change someone's sexual preference.

In many societies, especially those most influenced by Western media, there is a widespread view of the way adolescents 'naturally' behave. In fact, although the physical changes of puberty and adolescence occur everywhere, the existence of a teenage way of life varies greatly from society to society. Whether adolescents enter into a teenage way of life depends more on the lifestyle of the friends they mix with than on the stage of physical puberty they have reached.

## 9.2.2 Finding out more about sexual problems

Sexual abuse is discussed in Section 14.4 and not in this section.

When a child is brought to the clinic with a problem concerned with sexual development, it is important that the health professional has a clear view of the range of normal sexual behaviour in the society in which she works. All the same, it is always relevant to enquire:

- What exactly is the sexual problem about which the parent or perhaps the adolescent is worried about?
- When did it begin and how often does it occur?
- Does the child feel guilt or distress about the problem, whatever it is?
- Why have they come now, at this point in time, to ask about the problem?
- What effect do they think will occur as a result of the problem?
- Do they think this problem is widespread among other boys and/or girls or do they think it is unusual?
- Is there any possibility that the child/adolescent is being sexually abused or is abusing others? Is there any sign of bruising or other trauma in the genital area? (Do not examine unless there are grounds for suspicion.)
- Has the parent/adolescent noticed any sign of a sexually transmitted disease, for example is there a discharge from the penis or vagina, or any lesion in this area? (Do not examine unless there are grounds for suspicion.)
- In the case of an adolescent girl, is she sexually active? If so, is she engaging in unprotected sex?
- Generally, what are the attitudes to sex and sexual behaviour in the family? Is sex something that is talked about from time to time, hardly ever, or never?

In areas where HIV/AIDS is prevalent, it may be appropriate, after explaining the implications and obtaining consent, to refer the child for a blood test (see Section 12.8).

Now, given the information you have obtained, try to understand how this particular child has developed a sexual problem. Then go on to work out a plan to help.

## 9.2.3 Helping children and adolescents with sexual problems

Management of suspected sexual abuse is dealt with in Section 14.4.

Any positive results of tests for sexually transmitted disease, including HIV/AIDS, will require treatment as laid down in local protocols (see Section 12.8).

For most other reasons for referral for a sexual problem, the health professional will be able to reassure the parent/child that the behaviour in question is quite normal. When providing reassurance, health professionals should:

- take care to use very simple language, using words for penis and clitoris that the child/parent will understand
- make sure they do not mock or humiliate the parent/child because they have not understood that the problem is part of normal behaviour
- provide additional information about sex and sexual behaviour that might otherwise be neglected; the opportunity for sex education, including contraceptive advice, should not be missed
- in the case of a pregnant girl, ensure as good antenatal care as possible; work out how the girl can be supported by her family during the pregnancy and after birth
- make sure the parent/child feels they can return to the health professional for advice on the problem, especially if they do not feel reassured.

Now make a list of the ways in which the health professional might be able to help Mandara and her mother.

## 9.3 Self-starvation (anorexia nervosa)

**Case 9.3**

Ekta is a 15-year-old girl brought to the clinic by her parents because she will not eat and is losing weight. She was a slightly plump girl until about a year ago when, in the company of two other girls at school, she went on a diet. One of the other girls failed to start the diet and the other lost a few pounds and then went off the diet and put all the weight that she had lost back on. But Ekta just carried on dieting. Her parents, who to begin with were quite pleased that she had gone on a diet, began to get worried when her periods stopped. They took her to a clinic thinking that maybe she had a serious physical problem but the doctor could not find anything wrong with her and told them not to worry. She was a normal, healthy girl. But the dieting continued and now she looks terribly thin. Her parents do not know how much she has lost but clearly it is a considerable amount. She has also started to exercise every day to lose even more weight. Now her parents and her older sister get angry with her when she refuses to eat her meals, but it makes no difference. Ekta is a very bright, conscientious girl who has always been at the top of the class. Everyone likes her because she is so helpful to other people, for example, visiting her sick grandmother every day to make sure she is all right. The health professional cannot find anything physically wrong with her except that she is very thin and has rather low blood pressure. She weighs 35 kg, very little for a girl who is 5' 6" (168 cm) tall. What can the health professional do?

### 9.3.1 Information about self-starvation (anorexia nervosa)

The problem begins most commonly in the mid-teens, but can begin before puberty. It used to be very rare in LAMI countries; however, with increasing exposure to television programmes and advertisements in which the ideal shape for a girl is extremely thin, the problem is becoming more common in these countries. It is ten times more common in girls than in boys, and girls are often high achievers, unusually conscientious, kind and helpful. Self-starvation usually occurs in older girls in their late teens or early 20s. It often responds well to CBT (see p. 7).

In anorexia or self-starvation, the onset of menstrual periods is delayed or, if they have started, periods stop when the girl has lost a significant amount of weight.

Girls who self-starve often see themselves as fat and ugly even though they are not. This gives them the drive to lose weight. They refuse to eat, saying they are not hungry. To lose more weight they often vomit food they have just eaten and exercise excessively, and/or use laxatives to cause diarrhoea. They may have episodes of binge eating when they consume too much food. Binge eating or bulimia nervosa may occur in the absence of anorexia nervosa.

The cause of self-starvation is usually unknown, but:

- the problem is exacerbated in societies exposed to Western media, with its emphasis on the thin ideal
- there may be a genetic predisposition in affected girls
- there may be a particularly vulnerable personality type: stubborn, obsessional and self-sacrificing
- there may be fears about growing into adulthood regarding bodily changes and increased independence
- communication within the family about feelings may be limited
- there may be serious conflict between the parents.

Associated depression and anxiety are common, and constipation often arises as a result of the small food and liquid intake. With or without treatment, although about half of girls recover, the problem may become chronic with lifelong concern about diet and thinness. A very small proportion of girls die as a result of self-starvation or suicide.

## 9.3.2 Finding out more about girls who are self-starving

Take a careful account from both the parents and the girl separately. Find out especially:

- When did the problem begin?
- What triggered it?
- Who is present at meal times?
- Is there any binge eating?
- Is there any vomiting after meals or use of laxatives?
- What approach are the parents taking when their daughter will not eat: are they angry and pressurising or accepting and passive?
- How much exercise is the girl taking?
- What has happened to menstruation?
- Is the girl depressed? Is it possible that food refusal arises from depression or is it probably the other way round?
- Are there any delusional ideas suggestive of schizophrenia?
- What sort of personality did the girl have before the problem began: obsessional, perfectionist?
- How do the parents get on?

It is important to find out how the girl feels about her appearance. You can ask questions such as 'How do you feel about the way you look?', 'What weight would you ideally like to be?' and 'How do you feel about the portions of food your mum puts on your plate?' It is important not to be judgemental even if the girl's answers reflect gross distortions.

Ask how the girl feels about her adolescent development, for example 'How do you feel about growing into a woman?' A history of sexual abuse may be relevant in some cases.

In addition, carry out a full physical examination. The most important part of this is establishing an accurate height and weight. It is preferable for the girl to wear simple plain clothing and ensure that she is not hiding heavy weights inside her clothing to disguise how little she weighs. You will need a chart to establish just how much below the expected weight for her height she is. Less than 85% of the expected weight is a matter for concern (see WHO growth charts, www.who.int/childgrowth/standards/en/).

Also, is there any dehydration? Very occasionally, self-starvation may be due to endocrine disorders such as hyperthyroidism, hypopituitarism, malabsorption syndromes or a brain tumour.

Now, given the information you have obtained, try to understand how this particular girl has become involved in a pattern of self-starvation. Then go on to work out a plan to help.

### 9.3.3 Helping children and young people who are starving themselves

If the girl is dehydrated (look for dry, inelastic skin) and has a very low blood pressure (less than 80/50 mmHg), she is at risk of dying. If this is the case she needs admission to hospital for intravenous fluids or nasal tube feeding, compulsorily if she refuses. If this is not possible, then she needs treatment at home and given drinks of water or nutritious broths until she is reasonably well hydrated.

Girls need to be told that they have a very serious condition and may die if they carry on dieting. In girls under 18, the best result is likely if parents are involved and are encouraged to be firm about eating. She should be given frequent, small meals, perhaps four to six times a day. The aim should be to put on 1.5–2.0 kg (3–4 lbs) a week until she is at least 90% of the expected body weight. More rapid weight gain than this is undesirable, as too rapid a gain is likely to be followed by an equally rapid loss. In fact, weight gain is often disappointingly slow.

The girl should be kept in the home initially. When she puts on weight she should be allowed a little more activity. It is unwise to tell girls that they are looking better when they put on weight. They often perceive this as being told they are fat and ugly. At the same time as there is this emphasis on putting on weight, the girl should, if possible, have the opportunity to talk about her fears, especially those of growing up.

Parents also need help to keep the problem in perspective. They should try to be firm even if their daughter becomes angry with them. They will probably need support from the health professional if they are to succeed in this. Once the girl has put on sufficient weight and her periods have started or re-started, there is such a high rate of relapse that the health professional will need to check on progress from time to time.

When there are significant family conflicts or relationship difficulties, and in cases where this is maintaining the symptoms, family intervention is an important component of the treatment programme.

Now make a list of the ways in which the health professional might be able to help Ekta.

## 9.4 Self-harm

**Case 9.4**

A 15-year-old girl rushed into a health clinic in a rural area to ask the health professional to come to her home straight away. She thought her father had swallowed some liquid and was dying. The health professional rushed to the small farm where the family lived but the man was beyond help. He had killed himself by swallowing a large quantity of liquid pesticide that had been left lying around. The girl told the health professional that she was supposed to be married this year. Her father had offered a good bride price but when the harvest failed he had to tell his daughter that it would not be possible for him to find the money and she could not be married. She had set her heart on marrying the boy with whom a marriage had been arranged. Her father was deeply upset he had not been able to meet the cost. He was very fond of his daughter. Now the girl said she blamed herself and felt like killing herself. What can the health professional do?

**Case 9.5**

Daniel was a 14-year-old boy who was brought half-conscious by his father to a health clinic in a shanty area of a large city. The father said that the previous evening he had had an argument with his son about staying out late and not going to school regularly. He thought Daniel was being bullied at school and that this was the reason why he sometimes did not go, but his father thought his son ought to be able to stand up for himself against the bullies and had not accepted this as an excuse. This morning he had discovered that Daniel was deeply asleep and there was a half-empty bottle of paracetamol beside him. He had thrown cold water over him and eventually Daniel had woken up and admitted to having swallowed 15 of the tablets because he wanted to die. What can the health professional do?

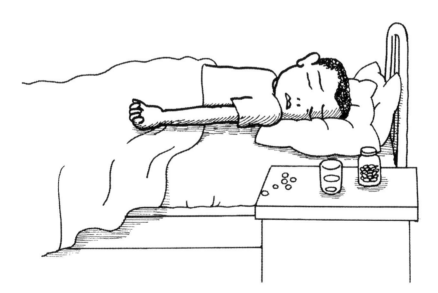

## 9.4.1 Information about self-harm

In many LAMI countries, suicide is an important cause of death in adolescents. The methods used depend on what is available. In rural areas, pesticides and poisonous domestic products are commonly employed. In urban areas, overdosing on tablets is increasingly used. Hanging occurs in both settings. Boys and girls are equally at risk of suicide.

Tablets are also most commonly used in non-fatal self-harming acts. Cutting or self-mutilation is another means of self-harming. Girls outnumber boys in self-harming that is non-fatal. The circumstances of both fatal and non-fatal self-harm are very variable. It may arise as:

- a sign of a chronic depressive disorder
- an impulsive, angry act arising from frustration, often in a young person with a history of aggressive behaviour
- a means of obtaining attention in a young person who feels neglected and unwanted
- a response to intolerable stress.

All suicidal thoughts and actions in children/adolescents should be taken seriously. They are usually a communication of desperation and a sign of limited problem-solving skills. If a child/adolescent has expressed suicidal thoughts, appraise the risk of a suicidal attempt. This will be greater if:

- the child has thought out how they would end their life
- they have actually taken steps to do this, such as getting a gun or buying poison or tablets
- they have marked depressive symptoms with distorted thinking
- they have shown violent, aggressive behaviour
- they have made a previous attempt.

In a young person who has self-harmed, the risk of repeated self-harm is greater if:

- the problem triggering the event has been present for more than a month
- the young person was alone in the house when he self-harmed
- the overdose was planned beforehand and was not an impulsive act
- the young person is still feeling hopeless about the future
- the young person was feeling sad for most of the time before the overdose
- measures were taken to avoid discovery
- a suicide note was left behind
- no attempt was made to obtain help after the suicidal act
- a violent or dangerous method was used.

Because of the risk of recurrence, all children/adolescents who have made a suicide attempt should be carefully assessed.

All children/adolescents with active suicidal thoughts or behaviour or who have recently made a suicide attempt should be carefully supervised by members of their family or friends. If the suicidal risk is serious, they should not be left alone at any time. At the same time, active steps should be taken to reduce the stress that has led to the self-harming behaviour.

## 9.4.2 Assessing children and adolescents who are at risk of self-harm or who have harmed themselves

The following approach can be used with children who are thought to be at risk of self-harm. If possible, they should be seen separately from their parents. After setting them at ease by talking about neutral subjects, you might go on to ask: 'What sort of things do you like doing with your friends? Do you still enjoy those things? What is it you've been most upset about recently?', and not 'Have you been upset about anything recently?', as this allows them to avoid talking about painful subjects.

'Do you sometimes think that people don't like you very much?', 'What makes you think that?'

'Do you feel you've done something bad?', 'What might that be?'

'How do you feel about the future?', 'Do you feel hopeless about what is going to happen to you?'

This may lead to questions probing suicidal thoughts and actions. These need to follow a progression moving from slight to serious suicidality:

'Have you felt at any time recently that really life isn't worth living?'

If answered positively: 'Do you mean that you have felt that you would be better off dead?'

If answered positively: 'Have you even thought of taking your own life?'

If answered positively: 'Have you even tried to take your own life?'

Again, if positive: 'When was that?', 'What did you do?', 'What happened?', 'Do you feel as bad as that now?'

The following questions might be used with children or adolescents who have recently self-harmed:

'You've obviously been feeling very upset recently. Please could you let me know what has been happening?'

'What was in your mind when you took the tablets?'

To help you decide what to do, you need to find out as much as you can about:

- whether the young person had emotional or behavioural problems before the attempt
- if so, whether these are still present
- how she gets on with other family members
- whether she has friends that can be confided in.

By asking the above questions you can find out whether the young person still has suicidal ideas.

In these circumstances, in order to make sense of the situation and decide on the risk of a further attempt, it is always necessary to see another family member. As well as finding out more about the information the young person has provided, it will be necessary to check on the amount of supervision it will be possible for the family to provide if suicidal ideas persist. If possible, talking to a friend and getting information from school would be helpful.

Now, using the information you have obtained from the young person and the family member(s) you have seen, try to understand what has happened and decide what is the best course of action.

### 9.4.3 Helping young people who have harmed themselves or attempted to do so

Once you have decided on the risk of self-harm, you need to discuss with the family how family members can protect the young person until the risk has reduced. Try to work out ways to reduce the stresses on the young person that have triggered the attempt or might trigger an attempt in the future. This may well involve contacting the school to talk to the young person's teacher.

Using the guidelines in other sections, try to treat any behaviour or emotional problems from which the young person is suffering. If possible, try to improve the communication in the family so that if the young person feels desperate again, he can talk about what is on his mind rather than communicating by self-harming.

Make it clear to the young person that you would be happy to see him if he is feeling desperate at any time in the future. Talk to family members about the importance of keeping safe all possible means of self-harm, such as pesticides, poisonous domestic products, firearms and dangerous medication.

# CHAPTER 10

# Alcohol and drug dependency

## 10.1 Alcohol problems

**Case 10.1**

Adut is a 17-year-old boy brought to the city clinic by his father at 10:00 h. His father had to support him as they walked in as Adut was staggering and hardly able to hold himself upright. Adut's father said that Adut had not got up to go to work that morning as usual. When his father went to his room to wake him, he realised he was drunk. He knew that Adut had come in very late the night before, well after his parents had gone to bed. Beside Adut's bed there were a number of cans of beer and an empty bottle of his mother's antidepressant tablets. It was clear that Adut had drunk a great deal of beer and swallowed some tablets. Fortunately, there had only been about ten tablets in the bottle. Adut worked in a bar. He was not really old enough to do this but he looked much older than his age. For the past few months Adut had often come home drunk. When he first started working at the bar a year ago everything was fine, but he began to see a girl older than himself who often came to the bar with men she had picked up. Adut had persuaded himself that she was in love with him and when she told him she did not want to go out with him, he became depressed and started to drink more heavily. While his father was telling this story Adut sat in a corner of the room, alternately vomiting and sobbing. What should the health professional do?

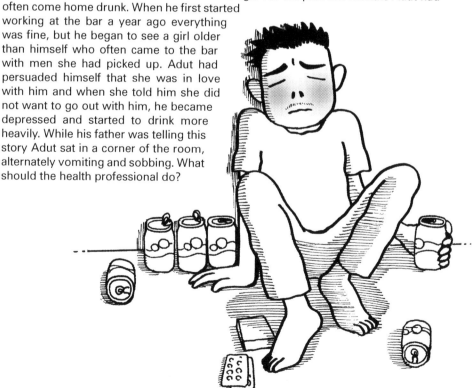

## 10.1.1 Information about alcohol problems

The sale of alcohol is legal in most countries, but the age at which the sale of alcohol becomes legal depends on the culture and the country. In countries in which the sale of alcohol to adults is legal, it is often easy for young people below the legal age to obtain alcohol. In many Muslim countries, however, drinking alcohol is not permitted for any section of the population.

Recommended limits of alcohol for young adults are 21 units a week for men and 14 units a week for women. A unit is one of the following:

- half a pint of beer – about 300 ml
- one small glass of wine – about 125 ml
- a small measure of spirits – about 30 ml.

Adolescents should drink less than this as their bodies are not capable of dealing with these levels without causing harm.

Young people drink alcohol to:

- experiment
- socialise with friends
- have fun or celebrate
- relieve boredom
- relax and remove inhibitions, for example in their sexual behaviour
- reduce worries, anxiety and depression.

Like other drugs, the effects of alcohol vary from person to person and how a young person may be affected may depend on:

- the quantity they have drunk
- how quickly they have drunk the alcohol
- whether they have mixed the alcohol with other drugs
- how regularly they drink
- their mood when they are drinking
- their age, gender and body weight
- their general health and nutrition
- whether they have been eating adequately while they were drinking alcohol
- whether they have been binge drinking (binge drinking means drinking heavily over a short period of time or drinking constantly over a number of days or weeks).

When drunk in small amounts, alcohol may make young people feel more relaxed; in larger amounts it may affect coordination and judgement and cause loss of consciousness. Other, more immediate effects of alcohol may include:

- feeling more confident
- feeling sleepy
- losing balance or feeling dizzy.

Short-term effects of drinking to excess include the following physical effects:

- a hangover
- nausea
- shakiness
- vomiting and memory loss
- injury
- alcohol poisoning.

Longer-term effects of heavy drinking over a period of time include:

- physical and psychological dependence on alcohol
- significant damage to the brain and liver
- risk of cancer of the mouth, throat or oesophagus
- possible increased risk of neurological disorders, heart problems and sexual problems (especially male impotence)
- emotional and mental health problems such as depression and anxiety
- problems at school, work and with relationships.

Being drunk affects the judgement of adolescents so that they risk:

- having unprotected or unwanted sex
- feeling bad about themselves and embarrassed by their actions
- losing friends or loved ones as a result of their behaviour
- spending money that is meant for more important items.

Using illegal drugs with alcohol is risky. If mixed with stimulants such as amphetamines, the young person may feel less drunk than he really is. If mixed with depressant drugs such as cannabis, there is a greater risk of passing out or overdosing.

In some cities both alcohol and illegal drugs are freely available if you have sufficient money. In these places young people may choose whether to spend an evening drinking alcohol or using illicit drugs, depending on what their friends are doing, how they want to feel and the cost.

Some young people who drink excessive amounts of alcohol are generally anti-authority and have been in trouble with the law. They frequently show aggressive, violent behaviour when they are drunk. Males especially may be involved in gang fighting or be physically abusive to their girlfriends.

Dependence or addiction to alcohol exists when a person feels physically ill if they stop drinking. This is called withdrawal syndrome. It is unusual for young people in their teens to develop alcohol dependence, but most adults who do develop such dependence started drinking alcohol heavily in their teens.

Drinking alcohol excessively damages physical and mental health. It may also result in the destruction of home life and in making serious study or regular employment impossible.

## 10.1.2 Finding out more about alcohol problems

Usually the young person with an alcohol problem will come to the attention of the police or a health professional because of accompanying emotional and behaviour problems, especially aggressive behaviour or fighting. These will need attention as described in other sections of this manual. Accidental injury is another common presentation.

- Obtain an account of how much alcohol the young person is consuming.
- Is the young person drinking alone or with others? If with others, is a heavy-drinking group the only one the young person belongs to?
- What needs are met by the drinking pattern – social (keeping up with the crowd) or psychological (relieving worry, anxiety or depression)?
- Ask about physical symptoms that might be alcohol-related such as gastritis.
- Ask about mental health problems such as anxiety and depression.
- Check on the presence of warning signs that the person is drinking too much, such as:
  - neglecting studies or work
  - getting into trouble over schoolwork or employment
  - feeling hungover in the morning

- thinking about alcohol a lot during the day
- feeling edgy
- drinking more alcohol than intended
- finding that more alcohol is needed to get the same effect.
- What are the family's attitudes to alcohol?
- What are the strengths of the young person's social position – at school, in employment, relationships with family and friends?
- Does the young person wish to change, cut down or stop his drinking?

Now, using the information you have obtained from the young person with an alcohol problem and the family member(s) you have seen, try to understand what has happened and decide what is the best course of action.

### 10.1.3 Helping young people with alcohol problems

Ask the young person what he hopes he will be doing when he is an adult. Then ask what he thinks will be the likely outcome if he carries on drinking at the same rate as he is now. Find out how much he wants to change. If he shows real motivation to change, then:

- decide with him whether to attempt to achieve complete abstinence or to aim for 'controlled drinking': abstinence is the preferred option, especially if the young person's health has already been affected
- if it is decided to achieve abstinence, then arrange a programme of alcohol withdrawal (Box 10.1)
- if it is decided to achieve controlled drinking, then use the tips in Box 10.2 to control the amount of drink used each day.

There may be little or no motivation to cut down drastically or stop drinking. This is usually the case with teenagers. In this situation advise on ways to make drinking safer (Box 10.2).

- Do not mix alcohol with other drugs
- Finish each drink – do not top up the current drink or you will not know how much you have drunk
- Know your limits – what may be fine for others may not be fine for you
- Do not drink and drive
- Stay with people you know and trust
- If you are having sex, use a condom to avoid the risk of a sexually transmitted infection or an unwanted pregnancy
- Try to develop friendships with others for whom drinking alcohol is not a necessary part of socialising

Whichever form of help is decided on there will be times when the young person goes through difficult times struggling to remain sober. The strategies in Box 10.3 may help the person through these times.

Now make a list of the ways in which the health professional might be able to help Adut.

Box 10.1  Alcohol withdrawal and its treatment

Alcohol withdrawal occurs when a person who is dependent on alcohol suddenly stops drinking. It usually begins within 24 hours of stopping drinking and lasts between 4 and 10 days. The more the person was drinking, the worse are the symptoms.

The common warning symptoms that a withdrawal reaction has started are:

- tremor
- shakiness
- poor sleep
- nausea
- anxiety
- irritability
- fever
- restlessness.

As the symptoms worsen, the person becomes confused, hallucinates and may have fits.

Treatment in the general healthcare setting should include:

- education about the relationship between the symptoms and the withdrawal from alcohol
- full physical examination (if the person has a fever, has fits, cannot drink fluids, is dehydrated or has a physical disorder, or is hallucinating or confused, refer them to a hospital)
- thiamine (a type of vitamin) – give 100 mg by intramuscular injection and prescribe a week's supply of thiamine tables (50 mg daily), multivitamins and folic acid (1 mg daily)
- a 4- to 6-day supply of chlordiazepoxide, to be taken as follows:
  - day 1, 25 mg four times a day
  - day 2, 25 mg three times a day
  - day 3, 25 mg twice a day
  - days 4 and 5, 25 mg at night
  - days 6 and 7, 12.5 mg at night
- alternatively, you can use diazepam, in the same way, starting from a dose of 5 mg four times a day.

Patel (2003)

Box 10.2  Controlled drinking

If a person chooses controlled drinking, then there are some tips you can suggest to control the amount of drink used every day.

- Keep track of how much you drink (if possible by recording it in a diary)
- Have at least 2 or 3 days in a week when you do not have any drink
- Alternate alcoholic drinks with non-alcoholic drinks
- Do not drink 'straight' alcohol – mix it with water or soda, so that one drink lasts longer
- Put less alcohol into each drink (e.g. drink only single pegs)
- Never drink in the daytime
- Make each drink last longer (e.g. an hour)
- Eat before you have your first drink
- Do not drink alcohol to quench your thirst; have water or other non-alcoholic drinks
- Reduce the time you spend in bars or with friends who drink heavily

Patel (2003)

Box 10.3 Dealing with difficult times while remaining sober

These are moments when it is especially difficult to stay sober. Suggest the following strategies to help the person to deal with such times.

- If you drink mainly at night, try to keep yourself busy, and go to places you cannot drink, such as a temple
- If you are in the habit of drinking with friends after work, try to organise a different social activity, such as going to see a film or do a sporting activity
- If you drink heavily only with certain friends, avoid these friends
- If you drink when alone, reduce the time you spend alone; for example, join a support group such as Alcoholics Anonymous or increase the time you spend with your family
- If you drink when you are under stress, learn ways of coping with stress and solving problems rather than blanking them out with alcohol

Patel (2003)

## 10.2 Drug problems

### Case 10.2

Adit is a 16-year-old boy whose father brought him to the clinic. For the past 6 months he has been one of a group of boys and girls of the same age smoking *charas* (cannabis). This group used to meet behind the sports stadium in the town where they lived. His father thought that Adit had been smoking *charas* quite heavily as he could smell it on his breath when he came home every evening. The father recognised the smell as he had smoked *charas* from time to time as a boy. Over the past few months Adit had become increasingly tired and lacking in energy. He had stopped going to the classes he had been attending in order to become an electrician. Instead, when he was not out with his friends, he would just sit in a chair and look at the ceiling. Then about a month ago he had started to behave strangely, muttering to himself. He did not seem able to think straight. When he talked, he did not make any sense. Then he began to accuse his mother of going through his clothes. He seemed really confused and at times almost delirious. His father had told him to stop going out with these friends, but he took no notice. What can the health professional do to help?

### 10.2.1 Information about drug problems

Illegal drugs are an important part of the youth culture that exists in many urban and some rural areas. Their use:

- makes young people feel that they are part of a group
- marks entry into the adult world
- reduces group anxiety
- results in a shared experience many young people find extremely enjoyable.

However, in some countries, illicit drugs have an important place in cultural or religious rituals. In these circumstances they are only taken on special occasions.

Illegal drugs can be extremely harmful to the individual, but unless health professionals understand the positive reasons why young people use them, they may not be in a good position to help when things go wrong.

Cannabis (hash, weed, grass, *bhang, charas, ganja*) is the illegal drug most widely used by young people. It is a depressant drug that produces a sense of relaxation and well-being. Occasional, experimental use of cannabis is not usually harmful. Excessive use may:

- result in apathy and a lack of motivation to get anything done
- trigger a brief state of confusion lasting a few hours
- trigger an episode of much longer-lasting schizophrenic psychosis in a vulnerable young person
- result in psychological but not usually physical dependence; if a regular user stops using cannabis, he really misses using the drug but does not usually have a physical withdrawal syndrome.

Other illegal drugs include amphetamines and 'ecstasy'. These are used because they give a 'buzz', with feelings of excitement and well-being. Excessive use of amphetamines may trigger acute psychosis. A number of deaths have been reported from the use of ecstasy as a result of overheating and dehydration.

Some groups of younger children, in their early teens or even younger, inhale solvents such as petrol, glue, lighter fluids and paint thinners. This gives them a sense of relaxation and well-being.

Heroin, cocaine, barbiturates and lysergic acid diethylamide (LSD) are used by a small minority of young people in some parts of the world. These drugs are generally regarded as more harmful than cannabis. The drugs are usually expensive, so young people who become 'hooked' on them have difficulty finding the money for their drug habit. In some countries, the use of 'crack cocaine' (a form of cocaine made by mixing powdered cocaine with baking powder and smoking it) is quite widespread among teenagers. All these drugs have serious harmful effects.

Young people who become addicted to alcohol or illegal drugs may take to crime, especially stealing from home and elsewhere, so that they can pay for their drug habit.

Although drug addiction is unusual in childhood and adolescence, most adult drug addicts began their drug habit in their teenage years.

## *10.2.2 Finding out more about young people who are using illegal drugs*

Usually the young person with a drug problem will come to the attention of the health professional because of being confused or because there are accompanying behaviour or emotional problems. They may be involved in stealing to obtain money to fund their drug habit or be depressed or showing signs of schizophrenia (see Section 11.2). They may have physical health problems, such as infections, due to the drug use or they may have run out of drugs and are having withdrawal symptoms.

Parents will often be the first people who want to help the young person. They may have noticed:

- the smell of cannabis
- that the young person has become secretive and refuses to communicate
- that he is always short of money and sums of money have started to go missing in the house.

You should ask parents:

- 'Have you noticed any change in his behaviour? Since when?'
- 'Do you suspect he is using drugs? If so, why?'
- 'How do you feel about this?' A sympathetic attitude could be helpful later on.

Occasionally, the young person may come for help because they have:

- an associated health problem
- run out of drugs and want the health professional to give them a supply
- withdrawal syndrome
- decided they really want to stop using drugs.

You should ask the young person:

- 'Which drugs are you using? How often do you take drugs?' This will tell you about the type and frequency of drug use.
- 'How do you take the drugs?' If by injection, ask: 'Do you share needles? If so, have you had a HIV test or hepatitis B test?'
- 'Have you tried to stop the drugs on your own? What happened?' Young people who have tried to stop may be more motivated to accept help.
- 'How is the habit affecting your health? Your relationships with other family members? Your studies or work?'
- 'Would you like to stop using the drugs? Why now?' Being motivated is an important sign that the person may succeed in giving up the habit.

Now, using the information you have obtained from the young person with a drug problem and the family member(s) you have seen, try to understand what has happened and decide what is the best best course of action.

## 10.2.3 Helping young people with drug problems

In most cases, young people using illegal drugs do not come to health professionals for help for their drug habit. They come because of an associated physical health problem, for example tiredness, depression, anxiety or signs of a psychotic illness. For advice on how to manage these problems, see the relevant sections.

If the young person is unconscious, has severe withdrawal or has a serious infection, then refer to a hospital emergency department. If the young person is not in need of urgent medical attention, then try and form a trusting relationship with him. Then:

- set a definite date for stopping taking the drug
- allow at least a week to recover from a withdrawal phase.

If there is a risk of serious withdrawal symptoms, then, if one is available, refer to a specialist drug clinic where drugs such as methadone can be used to reduce withdrawal symptoms.

The principles for treating the minority of drug users who are willing to receive treatment are abstinence, relapse prevention and rehabilitation. This requires a specialist facility. For young people who are not willing to stop now:

- refer to a community group that helps drug users
- consider ways of reducing the drug misuse, for example from smoking half a gram of heroin a day to a quarter of a gram
- move from more dangerous to less dangerous ways of using drugs, for example from injecting drugs to smoking them
- give advise on reducing the risk of infections from injections using dirty needles
- point out the damage that the drugs are causing
- always offer the young person a chance to come back to talk to you.

Now write down ways a health professional might be able to help Adit.

# CHAPTER 11

# Psychotic disorders

Psychotic disorders are unusual in childhood and adolescence but are serious when they occur. They consist of:

- bipolar disorder (severe mood swings); this used to be called manic–depressive psychosis
- delusions (false ideas without any basis in reality), hallucinations (sensory perceptions such as hearing voices when there is no one there) and disorders of thinking. These are most likely to be signs of schizophrenia, which may take different forms. All are serious, but there are now effective treatments for schizophrenia.

## 11.1 Bipolar disorder

**Case 11.1**
Indira was a 14-year-old girl brought to see a health professional by her mother. Her mother said that she had had to drag Indira to the clinic because she had not wanted to come and thought there was nothing wrong with her. Indira thought that she had never felt better. But for the past 3 months she had become more and more difficult and impulsive. She talked much more than normal and it was hard to interrupt her once she started. She got very angry when she was interrupted. She had been stealing money from her mother's purse and spending it on clothes she could not possibly afford. She was sleeping much less, only about 5 hours a night. Indira had never behaved like this before. She had always been a rather shy girl. About 2 years ago she had gone through a period of 6 months when she was sad and miserable and did not want to go out. It had never been clear why she was so depressed at this point. Indira's father had left home some years ago, after having relationships with a number of other women. He did not keep in touch. Indira has no brothers or sisters. What should the health professional do?

### 11.1.1 Information about bipolar disorder

People with bipolar disorder do not understand that they have a mental illness – they lack insight. It is called bipolar disorder because many people experience unusually elevated and depressed states for periods of time. Some people only have episodes of unusual happiness or irritability. The illness does not usually start before mid-adolescence.

Before the illness begins, the child or teenager may have shown mood swings more so than other children. There is usually a trigger, a stress, especially a loss, that triggers the illness. Symptoms in the 'manic' phase include:

- mood: feeling extraordinarily happy for no good reason, irritability

- thinking: believing that one is a very special, powerful person – handsome, good-looking, rich or having special abilities
- behaviour: rapid speech, overactivity, impulsive, lacking self-control (e.g. sexually), spending extravagantly, needing less sleep, drinking alcohol excessively or using drugs
- imagining things: hearing voices or seeing visions when there is nothing there.

In a manic phase it may be difficult to know whether bipolar disorder is present or whether the problem is mainly one of overactivity and lack of concentration. If the problem has been present from the early years and the child does not have mood swings, it is probably best to think of the illness as an attention disorder. If there are mood swings and the illness develops in adolescence, it is better to think of it as bipolar disorder. Children who have attention problems in earlier childhood may, however, develop bipolar disorder in later life.

In the depressed state the patient may show:

- great sadness
- false ideas of being guilty for something trivial or something he has not done
- poor sleep or excessive sleep
- poor appetite or eating too much
- lack of energy
- hopelessness about the future
- thinking about death and possibly suicide.

The illness is episodic. Each episode may last for weeks or months, but only rarely more than 2 years. There are also periods lasting months or years when the patient is well and without symptoms. In some episodes the patient may show signs of both unusual happiness and depression – this is a mixed form of the illness. Often someone else in the family has had a similar disorder. There may be a strong genetic influence.

Without treatment (see Appendix 2) to prevent further episodes, the illness can often be life-long.

## 11.1.2 How to assess bipolar disorder

- Check when the problem began. Did the child have mood swings even before the illness began? Did the child have any problems in attention and concentration before the illness began?
- What are the main features of the child's mental state? Is the child displaying an unusually cheerful mood, overactivity, irritability, false ideas about being wealthy or very bright, sleep disturbance, rapid speech, lack of self-control, or extravagant spending? Has the child ever been very sad, had ideas of being guilty of something quite trivial, or been constantly tired and lacking in energy?
- Was there a stressful event, a loss, when the episode of unusual cheerfulness and overactivity began?
- How has the child's life been affected by the illness at home or at school? Is the child in trouble at school or with the police for antisocial behaviour? Is the child able to concentrate on schoolwork?
- Has anyone else in the family had a similar problem?
- If the child or adolescent is in a depressed state or has been in such a state recently, are there any suicidal ideas or is the child at risk of taking his own life?

Now, using the information you have obtained from the young person with bipolar disorder and the family member(s) you have seen, try to understand what has happened and decide what is the best course of action.

## 11.1.3 Helping young people with bipolar disorder

If the diagnosis is definite, then the mainstay of treatment is antipsychotic medication (see Appendix 2). Because of side-effects to which the young are especially sensitive, begin with a small dose and build up gradually.

It is really important that the medication is taken regularly, so parents should be involved in making sure this happens. Patients with this condition are often not cooperative as they lack insight and think that there is nothing wrong with them. At the same time, patients should be protected from getting involved in risky and perhaps dangerous behaviour. Any money at home should be securely put away so that the child cannot steal and spend it. Someone should escort the child everywhere to prevent him from getting into trouble for sexually inappropriate or other risky behaviours.

If the child goes into a depressive state, the possibility of suicidal behaviour should be borne in mind. Again, a close eye needs to be kept on the child to prevent self-harm (see Section 9.4). If the child's problem becomes chronic and he develops repeated episodes of unusual happiness and depression, a mood stabiliser should be prescribed (see Appendix 2).

When in a stable state, the child needs to be helped to avoid stresses that might trigger another episode. Other family members need to be involved in the management of the disorder, as they can play a very helpful part in keeping the patient well.

Now make a list of the ways in which the health professional might be able to help Indira.

# 11.2 Schizophrenia

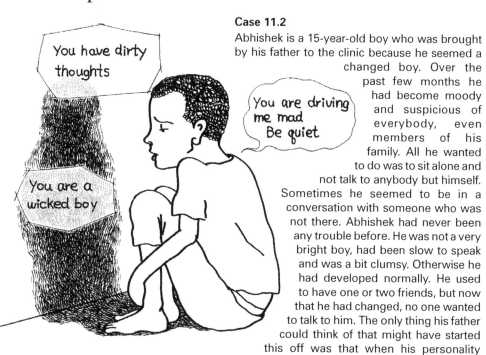

Case 11.2
Abhishek is a 15-year-old boy who was brought by his father to the clinic because he seemed a changed boy. Over the past few months he had become moody and suspicious of everybody, even members of his family. All he wanted to do was to sit alone and not talk to anybody but himself. Sometimes he seemed to be in a conversation with someone who was not there. Abhishek had never been any trouble before. He was not a very bright boy, had been slow to speak and was a bit clumsy. Otherwise he had developed normally. He used to have one or two friends, but now that he had changed, no one wanted to talk to him. The only thing his father could think of that might have started this off was that when his personality began to change he was smoking a good deal of *bhang* (cannabis). His father did not like him doing this but as he had smoked *bhang* himself when he was younger he could not really say very much about it. Abhishek's father wondered whether he was turning out to be like his wife's brother. This man had become very odd at the age of 19 and was in a mental hospital. What should the health professional do?

## 11.2.1 Information about schizophrenia

As with bipolar disorder, people with schizophrenia lack insight and do not understand that they have a mental illness. In schizophrenia, there may be several problems.

1   Thinking problems
    i     The patient may have difficulty in thinking clearly and logically.
    ii    He may think that his thoughts are being interfered with.
    iii   He may have delusions – beliefs that are not true, such as that people are all against him.
    iv    The delusion that everything that is happening in the world is somehow aimed at him. So, for example, he may believe that programmes on the television refer to him, or that others are talking about him.
    v     The patient may have a strange belief that there is something odd going on in his body, for example that there is an animal inside his belly.
2   Mood problems: the patient may find it difficult to express emotions or feel empty of emotions.
3   Behaviour problems
    i     Withdrawal from usual activities
    ii    Restlessness
    iii   Aggressive behaviour
    iv    Odd behaviour such as hoarding rubbish
    v     Not washing or cleaning himself properly
4   Problems of perception
    i     Seeing things that are not there (visual hallucinations)
    ii    Hearing voices when there is no one present (auditory hallucinations). The voices may accuse the patient of things he has not done. Sometimes the patient will talk to these voices. He cannot get them out of his head.

There may also be symptoms of depression or mania (see Section 11.1.1) – this is known as schizoaffective disorder.

Schizophrenia may begin at any time but most commonly it begins in the mid- to late teens or early 20s. Sometimes it starts for the first time much later in life. It may begin gradually or very suddenly. In some individuals, the illness may last for a short period of time and not recur, while in others the course can be chronic. There is sometimes a period lasting weeks or months in which the patient is very disturbed and agitated and has a number of upsetting, false beliefs. This may be followed by a period when the patient is much less disturbed but has little energy and finds thinking difficult. This may last for months or years before another episode of acute disturbance. This cycle may go on for the whole of the patient's life.

Language is slow to develop in early life in some patients who later develop schizophrenia. They may always have had difficulty in making friends and been rather isolated.

Schizophrenia is thought to be caused by physical changes in the brain, however it may begin after a stressful event. Smoking cannabis (*bhang*, weed, grass, hemp) may trigger an episode of schizophrenia in people who are likely to get it regardless. Quite often there is someone else in the family who has had schizophrenia. There is a strong genetic influence.

## 11.2.2 Finding out more about a child who may have schizophrenia

*   Check when the problem began. Has the patient always had problems making friends and getting on with other people or is this something new?
*   Were there any upsetting events occurring at the time the illness began? Was the patient smoking *bhang* (cannabis)?

- What symptoms has the child shown? Check for disturbances of thinking, including the presence of false beliefs. Does he think that his thoughts are being interfered with? Has the patient been talking to himself as if there is someone there when there is not? Does the patient behave as if he is seeing things when there is nothing there? Has the patient's behaviour been odd in any way? Are there any signs of depression?
- Does anyone else in the family have any signs of mental illness?
- How is the patient's life affected by the illness? Has he been able to go to school or work?
- Have the lives of other members of the family been affected in any way? For example, does someone have to look after the patient in case he wanders off or hurts someone?

Now using the information you have obtained from the young person with schizophrenia and the family member(s) you have seen, try to understand what has happened and decide what is the best course of action.

## 11.2.3 How to help a child or adolescent who may have schizophrenia

If the diagnosis is definite, then the mainstay of treatment is antipsychotic medication (see Appendix 2 for details). Because young people are more sensitive to medication side-effects, begin with a small dose and only build up gradually. It is really important that the medication is taken regularly, so parents should be involved in making sure this happens. Patients with this condition are often not cooperative as they lack insight and think that there is nothing wrong with them. It is important to remember that medication is likely to shorten the acutely disturbing part of the illness but it is not likely to be a cure. The patient may well need medication for the rest of his life.

At the same time as being given the medication, the patient should be given the opportunity to talk about what is upsetting him. The health professional should not argue with the patient or try to persuade him that his false beliefs are wrong. It may be helpful to try to get the patient to check the evidence for his beliefs. For example, if he thinks that everything on television refers to him, you could ask whether anything might make him think this was not the case.

Family members also need to have the opportunity to learn about schizophrenia. It is helpful for them to know that it is thought to be a disease caused by physical changes in the brain. Although stress may bring the illness on, this is not the main reason the patient has developed the illness. Family members may need help to cope with the patient, especially if he wanders off or is aggressive.

Patients with schizophrenia may need looking after for the rest of their lives; but with medication, it may be possible for them to be independent and look after themselves and even return to study or work.

Now make a list of the ways in which the health professional might be able to help Abhishek.

CHAPTER 12

# Chronic physical illness and disability

Mental health problems in children and adolescents may be linked to physical illnesses, including diabetes mellitus, asthma, eczema, congenital heart disease and HIV infection. However, there is a closer link between mental health problems and disorders affecting the brain, such as epilepsy and cerebral palsy, than there is with other physical conditions.

## 12.1 Physical illness and mental health

**Case 12.1**

Lakshmi is a 9-year-old girl well known to the local primary healthcare professional because she has chronic asthma. The health professional has learned over the past 3 years since the diagnosis of asthma was made that understanding Lakshmi's mental health and the social conditions in which she lives has been really important in keeping her alive and able to go to school. Some of Lakshmi's asthma attacks come on when she has a cold or the flu or when she has been exposed to pollen in the spring. Some of her worst attacks are triggered by excitement and disappointment. Helping her parents to prevent Lakshmi getting too excited at the time of festivals and present-giving has reduced her attacks. A year ago, Lakshmi started to refuse to go to school because she was worried about having an attack there. The health professional was able to talk to the teachers to explain what should be done if Lakshmi had an attack in school and this reassured the teachers so that she was able to attend regularly. Lakshmi's family lives in an overcrowded shack in a poor part of the city. There is nothing that the health professional can do about the living conditions, but she was able to help her mother and father to stop smoking so that the air at home was less polluted and there was more money to spend on food. Now Lakshmi has started to be very disobedient and does not want to take the medication that seems to prevent the attacks. The health professional will have to try to understand this non-adherence with treatment and also help Lakshmi understand why it is important for her to take her medication regularly if it is to help.

Of course not all children who attend primary care clinics have such a rich set of links between their physical illness and their mental health and social circumstances as described in the case above, but many children have at least one of these features.

### 12.1.1 Information about physical illness and mental health

Chronic physical illness is common. About one in five children are affected by conditions such as asthma, eczema, diabetes, spinal deformities, heart conditions and tuberculosis. Children with a physical illness have about twice as many mental health problems as other children in the population. Certain physical illnesses have a much higher rate of associated mental health problems. These include epilepsy and other conditions affecting brain function.

There is no particular type of mental health problem linked to physical illness, although children with illness affecting the brain have a particularly high rate of difficulties with activity, attention and concentration. Sometimes the mental health problems arise directly from the illness, for example a child with a brain tumour might be depressed on learning of his prognosis. Often mental health problems are triggered by stresses, such as parental mental illness, that might be experienced by all children regardless of whether they have a physical illness or not.

Cultural influences affect the way parents and children themselves see their illness. This has implications for treatment. For example, if the parents of a child with a curvature of the spine believe that their child has been bewitched, this will affect the way the health professional talks to them about the ways in which the child might be helped.

Chronic physical illness may have an effect on the self-esteem of children. They may think that they are not worth bothering about, that it would be better if they had not been born or, to the contrary, they may feel special and pleased that they get so much attention. All this will affect their likelihood of becoming, for example, depressed, anxious or aggressive. In addition, parents react in many different ways to having a child with a chronic physical illness. For example, some parents are brought closer together by having a shared problem to face and deal with. With other parents, the child's illness may lead to arguments, even to separation and divorce.

The care of a child with a physical illness is likely to involve extra expense, for example in buying medicines or taking time off work to bring the child to a health clinic or hospital. The health professional should bear this in mind when counselling parents. The lives of brothers and sisters of a child with a chronic illness are often affected. They may be very caring or resentful. This will have an impact on family life that parents may find it helpful to discuss.

Some children with acute or chronic physical problems may need admission to hospital, usually for short periods but sometimes for weeks at a time. In LAMI countries, virtually all children admitted to hospital are accompanied by an adult, usually a parent or other relative. Most children are upset, at least to some degree, by having to come into hospital. If possible, admissions should be avoided by investigating and treating children as out-patients.

## 12.1.2 Principles of mental healthcare in children with physical illness

- Try to be alert to the ways in which the mental health of children with a chronic illness may be affecting the illness and the approach you should take in assessment and management.
- Listen to all the concerns parents express about their child with a physical illness. Sometimes these concerns may not be about the illness itself but may be even more important than treating the illness.
- Before you talk to children and parents about what might be the cause of an illness and how it might be managed, always find out from them what their ideas are and what they have already tried.
- If at all possible, try to see both parents (if available) at least from time to time. This will help communication between the parents.
- If parents or children get upset when you see them, show them that you understand how they feel and are prepared to share their pain (e.g. 'I know how hard this is for you'), rather than changing rapidly to another subject.
- Try to learn about the child's social circumstances. For you, the child's problem will, rightly, come first. However, it helps to understand a mother's apparent disinterest in her

child's condition if you know that her main concern is for her husband to stop beating and sexually abusing her when he comes home drunk every night.

- Keep in mind that a large part of a child's life is spent in school. The signs of illness and behaviour in school may be very different from that at home. If possible, get to know the local school and keep in touch with teachers about children with a chronic physical illness. They may have very useful information to give you. With the parent's permission, you can provide information to them that may enable them to give the child a better experience in school.

- Try to help parents feel that they are doing a good job looking after their child. It is very easy for parents to feel that they are failures. Give praise wherever you can, even for care that seems to you rather minimal, especially if you have seen at least some improvement.

- As with children with a physical disability, know what is available locally that might help families with a child with a chronic illness. If there are other parents with a child with a similar problem, consider putting them in touch with each other so that there can be some mutual help and support.

- If parents and/or children are not following treatment instructions, try to understand why this is happening rather than just telling them off. Understanding sometimes leads to change, while telling off rarely produces adherence – more commonly it results in resentment and even less adherence.

- When children are admitted to hospital in LAMI countries, they are nearly always admitted with an accompanying adult, usually a parent or other relative. All the same, a hospital admission is likely to be an upsetting experience for the child. The following measures will help to reduce distress.

  - Parents should prepare young children for admission to hospital by telling them stories about other children admitted to hospital and reading such stories from books.

  - Parents should never threaten children with admission to hospital if they are naughty.

  - If an admission is planned, then the child might be able to visit the ward and meet the staff before being admitted so that it will not be so strange to him later on.

  - If an emergency admission is necessary, this will be easier if the parents have explained about hospitals to the child beforehand. Emergency admission is so common that parents should educate their children about hospitals in cases where hospitalisation is anticipated or may be necessary.

  - Children should be prepared for all unpleasant procedures in a way suitable for their age. Children should not be given procedures without any warning.

  - Nursing and medical staff should be trained in working with children and in understanding how children react to stress.

  - If possible, children should have nurses allocated to them so that they become familiar with two or three members of staff and learn to trust them.

  - The organisation of the ward routine should be child-centred and not arranged for the convenience of the staff.

  - As far as possible, the food provided should be what the child is familiar with.

- Working with very sick children is very stressful. This should be generally understood, and young, inexperienced staff should be encouraged to talk to their seniors about how they are feeling about their work.

- Parents should expect their children to be upset when they are discharged from hospital, however good the care has been. They should be prepared to give their children extra attention at this time.

## 12.2 Physical disability

**Case 12.2**

An 8-year-old boy, Dilip, was carried to the clinic by his mother to see the health professional because of an eye infection. Although the health professional thought she knew most of the people living in the community she served, she had never seen Dilip before. She had seen his mother but did not know of Dilip's existence. Dilip had been unable to move his legs from about the age of 18 months after contracting meningitis that had left him brain-damaged. It turned out that Dilip's mother was deeply ashamed of having a son with a disability. It had taken a lot of courage for her to walk to the clinic carrying her son in front of her neighbours, but she had been worried he would lose his sight so she had had to come. The health professional prescribed some drops for Dilip's eyes and reassured the mother that the infection would be cured in a short time. She talked to Dilip and found that he also seemed to have some learning problems. He had never been to school and had been looked after entirely at home. The health professional wondered whether she could do anything to help in addition to prescribing the eye drops.

### 12.2.1 Information about physical disability in children

Physical disability is relatively common in children living in LAMI countries. The exact frequency is not known, but in many areas about 2 in every 100 children have a disability severely affecting their movements. Physical disability may show itself in a variety of ways:

- impairment of movement
- visual impairment
- hearing impairment
- intellectual impairment, specific or general intellectual disability
- a combination of the above – this is common; for example, cerebral palsy may be accompanied by intellectual disability.

Although in high-income countries most physical disability is caused by genetic disease, in LAMI countries infection is the most common cause. Poliomyelitis, tuberculosis and meningitis are the most common infections producing physical disability. In some areas, HIV/AIDS is also a significant cause. Cerebral palsy or the inability to move one or more limbs as a result of brain damage is also relatively frequent. This may be due to a genetic disease, injury during pregnancy, at birth or early in life, head injuries or infection.

Parents often think that their child has a physical disability because of witchcraft or other causes related to their religious beliefs.

Infectious disease is linked to poverty and poor social conditions, so physical disability is more common among disadvantaged groups. Parents and other caregivers are often financially stretched, with very little support, either material or emotional.

A high proportion of children with physical disability do not go to school. They are also often excluded in other ways, socially isolated and stigmatised. This may be related to the shame their parents experience.

Children with a physical disability may receive poor healthcare and have low rates of immunisation. They may be neglected at home, with care passed on to elderly grandparents or servants who ill-treat them.

Children with a physical disability have a high rate of mental health problems, occurring at least twice as frequently as in children without such disabilities.

Access to aids that would make a great difference to their lives, such as wheelchairs, prostheses and hearing aids, is often limited. When support is available, it is more likely to be provided by charitable organisations than by the government.

All this should not obscure the fact that some children with a physical disability are well looked after, have good healthcare, have access to the aids they need, attend school and lead happy and fulfilled lives.

Now, given the information you have obtained, try to understand how the physical disability is affecting the life of this particular child. Then go on to work out a plan to help.

## 12.2.2 What the health professional can do to help children with a physical disability

To begin with, health professionals need to make their own observations as well as to find out from the parents and child the following.

- Is the child well cared for? Is there evidence of neglect or physical abuse such as bruising?
- Is the child getting good healthcare? Has the child been immunised?
- Is the child in school? If not, why not?
- Has the child access to aids that might make a difference to his quality of life, such as a wheelchair, prosthesis (artificial limb), hearing aid or spectacles?
- Is the mother getting help from her family or from the community?
- Is there a voluntary organisation that might be able to help with financial support, counselling or aids to daily living, such as handrails and ramps?
- Does the child have a mental health problem? Children with brain damage are particularly likely to have attention and concentration problems, but they may also have significant depressive feelings and anxiety, or behaviour problems.

Having assessed the situation, the health professional may be able to help in a number of ways.

- Carefully check all aspects of heath and disability, as simple treatable problems are often easily missed in children with a disability. For example, treating constipation, providing appropriate spectacles, ensuring good dental health and good hearing, and treating epilepsy can often greatly improve a child's quality of life, even when only supportive treatment is available for the main disability.
- Give advice on nutrition and hygiene; without such information, it may be difficult for the parents to manage.
- If the child is not in school, check why this is and whether there is a way in which he might attend, even if only part time.
- Check on the health status of the child and, for example, ensure he is up to date on immunisations.
- If it seems as if the child's mobility or sensory abilities could be improved, put the parents in touch with a charitable foundation that could be helpful in the provision of aids or financial support.
- If the child has a mental health problem, give advice as suggested elsewhere in this manual, depending on the nature of the problem.
- Talking to influential people in the community about ways in which the parents might be helped to feel less stigmatised and more included in community life.
- Put the parents in touch with other parents who have a child with a physical disability so that they can find mutual support.

## 12.3 Hearing impairment

**Case 12.3**

Rahul was a 7-year-old boy who was brought to the health professional by his father, who said his son was always in trouble at school for being naughty and not paying attention. The health professional talked to Rahul and noticed that the boy seemed to be paying close attention to her lips when she spoke. She turned the boy round and asked him in a quiet voice to put his finger on his nose. The boy did not move. She then turned the boy to face her and made the same request. The boy did as he was told. What should the health professional do?

### 12.3.1 Information about children with poor hearing

Hearing impairment in a child may be mild to severe, depending on the amount (measured in decibels) of hearing loss. Deafness can be caused by:

- a problem of conduction of sound through the external (outer) or middle ear: this usually produces mild to moderate deafness. It is most commonly due to wax blocking the outer ear and chronic middle-ear effusion – serous otitis media (infection in the middle ear or 'glue ear');
- sensorineural damage: the nerves carrying impulses from the ear to the brain may be affected by genetic conditions or by damage resulting from viral infection of the fetus, especially by cytomegalovirus or rubella;
- damage to the cochlea (the inner ear where sounds are turned into electrical impulses that go to the brain): this can happen after a child has had meningitis and can also be due to drugs such as antimalarials and aminoglycosides, as well as persistent loud noise.

The most important effect of hearing impairment is on language development (see Section 4.2). Even mild hearing loss may result in delayed language development. Poor language development may lead to learning and reading difficulties.

Behaviour may also be affected. Children who cannot understand instructions because they cannot hear them are likely to become frustrated. This may result in:

- temper tantrums and disobedience
- problems of attention and distractibility (which may seem like ADHD, although rarely children may have both conditions)
- emotional problems with anxiety or depression
- social difficulties in mixing with other children.

### 12.3.2 Finding out about children with hearing impairment

Children born with poor hearing need to be identified as soon as possible after birth. It is possible to diagnose hearing loss accurately in babies shortly after birth, but this requires expensive equipment. Such equipment (otoacoustic emissions and automated auditory brain stem response) will not be readily available to most health professionals working in primary care. In a small number of centres in LAMI countries, all babies are screened using such equipment, sometimes in association with the local immunisation programme.

Without such equipment it is possible to obtain a reasonably good idea whether a child aged between 7 and 9 months has hearing loss by asking the mother whether the infant turns his head in the direction of speech or noises and whether he reacts with a startle response to sounds such as clapping behind his ears. The health professional can try making a quiet noise, with, for example, a rattle, behind the child's head when the child's attention is engaged elsewhere and observing whether the child's head turns. However, even if the child turns its head, it may have done so for other reasons and still be deaf. If there is any doubt about the child's hearing, the child should be observed and retested when a little older. In cases of doubt, if at all possible the child should be referred for more detailed testing. If the mother expresses any concerns about her child's hearing, they should be taken very seriously. Parents are usually accurate when they suspect deafness.

With older children, aged 3 years or more, a more accurate diagnosis can be made even without expensive equipment, if the child does not have significant intellectual disability. The health professional should cover their mouth with a sheet of paper and taking care to look only at the child's eyes, give a simple command such as 'Show me your nose'. A normal child should be able to respond accurately and quickly at the lowest voice level when the examiner is about a metre away. A child who does not turn his head to a whisper behind him is likely to have mild hearing impairment. Lack of response to a normal voice means that there is probably moderate impairment. A child who does not respond to a loud voice probably has severe impairment.

If a child is deaf, examination of the child's eardrum may show the ear canal to be full of hard wax, a dull yellow eardrum if there is fluid behind it or a red eardrum if there is infection. A child who has had many ear infections may have a perforation (hole) in the eardrum, although these examinations need some practice and skill. Most conductive losses are mild or moderate. Children with sensorineural deafness more often have severe hearing loss. In all children with developmental, behaviour or emotional problems, the possibility of hearing loss should be considered. If there is any possibility of hearing impairment, this should be investigated with the best available equipment.

It is particularly difficult to diagnose or rule out deafness in some children with ASD as they are unresponsive to sounds most of the time. They are, however, very likely to pay attention and even become agitated when they are exposed to unfamiliar sounds. Some children with ASD, especially those for whom congenital rubella is responsible, are likely to have an associated hearing impairment.

Sometimes children with only moderate hearing problems have the greatest behaviour and emotional problems because the hearing difficulties have gone unnoticed – they know others are talking to them or possibly about them but cannot communicate this and can become very upset or appear disobedient.

Now, given the information you have obtained, try to understand how this child's hearing problem has arisen and is affecting his life. Then go on to work out a plan to help.

### 12.3.3 Helping children with hearing impairment

If, from the information provided by the family and from observation, it seems likely that the child does have a hearing impairment, then if at all possible the child should be referred for more expert diagnosis and advice on treatment. If no expert advice is available, and it is not possible for the child to be fitted with a hearing aid, then the following measures should be taken.

1   Treat the cause. This is not likely to be possible with sensorineural deafness, but an infection in the middle ear may be treatable with antibiotics or simple surgical procedures if someone with specialist surgical expertise is available in the area. Wax in the external ear can be gently and carefully removed. This is best done by putting 2 or 3 drops of warm vegetable oil in the ear daily for about 2 weeks.

2   Make family members and school teachers aware of the hearing loss. If mild or moderate hearing loss is present, they will need to speak more clearly and ensure that the child can

see them easily when they are talking. Background noise should be kept to a minimum. In severe hearing impairment, they will need to develop sign language with the child.

3   Any associated developmental (especially language), behaviour and emotional problems should be managed as described in the relevant sections.

4   Children whose language is delayed because of mild or moderate hearing impairment should be helped to communicate using every possible means. Further, it should not be assumed that because their language is delayed they lack intelligence. Their abilities in manual tasks not involving language should be noted and encouraged.

Now write down what the health professional can do to help Rahul.

## 12.4 Visual impairment

**Case 12.4**

Ajit is 2 years old when his mother brings him to the clinic because he does not seem to understand simple requests like her other children did at his age. She has not brought him to the clinic before. The health professional notices not only that Ajit's development is more like that of a 1-year-old, but that he does not seem to look around or notice anything that is going on around him. What should the health professional do about his possible visual problem?

### 12.4.1 Information about children with limited sight or lack of sight

Visual problems in children are often present from birth or develop in early childhood. Some are caused by genetic defects, as a result of damage to the baby's brain around the time of birth or because of an infection picked up in the womb or shortly after birth. The most common causes of blindness are vitamin A deficiency, measles, conjunctivitis in the newborn, congenital cataract, and retinopathy of prematurity. If a baby is born blind, it is sometimes only recognised several weeks after birth when it is noticed that his eyes do not follow a moving object such as a face, or the baby is very late to smile in response to the mother's face. Most, but by no means all, children with visual problems that have been present from birth also have some degree of intellectual disability. They are often slow in their motor, language and social development. Although onchocerciasis or 'river blindness' and trachoma are common causes of blindness in adults, visual problems are not usual in children with these infections.

Children who are blind usually have roving eye movements and do not appear to focus on anything. Children with poor sight often have a squint or lazy eye where the eyes do not move together so that the child may be seen to be looking with only one eye. Older children with visual problems (nystagmus, paralytic squints) may also look at things at an unusual angle. Severe visual problems in children are also associated with:

*   various habits or mannerisms not seen in other children, such as rocking, eye pressing, repetitive noises and flapping their hands in front of their eyes
*   a high rate of behaviour and emotional problems, especially anxiety disorders.

Some of the additional difficulties in children with visual impairment from birth are caused by physical damage or poor function of the brain or visual pathways. However, some difficulties are environmental and open to change.

*   Lack of appropriate stimulation. The usual types of stimulation provided to children will not help the development of a child with visual impairment. Stimulation and games involving touch and sound need to be encouraged.

- Depression in other family members, especially the mother who may be very upset and possibly blames herself for her child's condition.

Later in childhood, it may become clear that a child's reading problem is caused by short- or long-sightedness. The child may be holding a book very close to his eyes or may only be able to watch the television if sitting very close to the screen.

Vitamin A deficiency is common in areas where diets are poor. Children can be affected from 1 year of age – the first signs are difficulty seeing in the dark (night blindness) and white spots on the sclera (whites of the eyes). Vitamin A supplementation for every baby and young child is important to help prevent this form of blindness in areas where this is a problem.

Measles can cause scarring of the cornea, especially in children with vitamin A deficiency. It is important to ensure all children are immunised against measles and any child with measles is correctly treated and has their eyes examined for corneal ulcers.

## 12.4.2 Finding out about children with visual impairment

- The baby may be brought to the health clinic because the mother suspects that her child cannot see. The baby may not seem to notice objects or be slow to smile or startle and seem surprised when the mouth is touched. The eyes of a baby that is blind often move rapidly from side to side.
- Visual impairment may be confirmed by passing a finger or a light in front of the baby and observing whether the eyes follow it. The baby may fail to blink when a hand is moved rapidly towards the face as if to strike it.
- As blindness is often caused by a genetic defect, babies suspected of being blind should be carefully examined for the possible presence of other genetic problems such as deafness and heart defects.
- Babies identified as visually impaired need careful developmental assessment (see Section 4.1) as they are likely to be delayed in other aspects of their development.
- A baby suspected of visual impairment needs referral to an specialist centre if one is available.
- A child over 1 year who has a squint should be referred to a specialist if one is available. The child may need spectacles and some children may be helped by an operation on the eye muscles to help the eyes move together.
- When an older child needs to hold a book close to their eyes or to get near to the television to watch programmes, the child's eyes will need testing. The child should go to the local optician, if available, to get prescription spectacles.
- Children with significant long sight, some of whom may have a squint, may find reading or studying tiring.
- A quick and easy way to check for eye-sight problems is by using the pinhole test. Punch a small hole in a paper card and ask the child to read while looking through the pinhole. If the child can see better through the pinhole, it is suggestive of problems with refraction. Note that children will often be able to see easily for most simple vision tests, so if it is possible, the child should have their eyes checked by an optician/optometrist.

Now, given the information you have obtained, try to understand how this child's visual problem has arisen and is affecting his life. Then go on to work out a plan to help.

## 12.4.3 Helping babies and children who are visually impaired

Babies who are blind or severely visually impaired need as much non-visual experience as possible. It is important to let them learn about the world by using their other senses, putting objects into their hands, and making sure they recognise objects by their feel and smell. Babies who cannot see their mothers and other family members are very likely to find separation from them more difficult. Babies and young children should be reassured when left alone, even for brief periods.

Family members should be encouraged to talk to babies who are visually impaired about things they cannot see, about what is happening to them and around them. Particular attention should be given to the encouragement of language development using other ways (see Section 15.4).

Children with visual impairment who develop anxiety problems should be treated as described in Section 7.3.3.

In older children with learning difficulties, vision should always be tested to check whether there is a need for spectacles.

What can the health professional do to help Ajit's visual problems?

# 12.5 Cerebral palsy

**Case 12.5**

Abhi is a 7-year-old boy brought to the clinic by his mother because he is not eating properly. The health professional has known Abhi since he was 6 months old. To begin with, he had developed normally, but after a few months his mother noticed that when he kicked his legs his right leg did not move as much as his left. He did not seem to use his right arm when he held things. The health professional had tested the power on his left side and found it was normal but his right arm and leg were definitely weak. Abhi was diagnosed with congenital hemiplegia. This is a type of cerebral palsy present from birth. It was not known why Abhi had this problem but his mother had had a small bleed when she was 7 months pregnant and it may have been that the left side of his brain had been deprived of oxygen and been damaged. Generally, Abhi was making good progress. He had been slow to walk but now was walking well, although with an obvious limp. He could even run without falling over. His speech had developed normally. He was a friendly boy.

Why was he not eating properly? It turned out that he was being teased at school where he was called 'Hoppy' by other boys because of the way he walked. At playtime when the boys chose sides to play football, Abhi was never chosen until right at the end, and then no one wanted him on their side. He was coming home miserable every afternoon and not wanting to eat his supper. What could the health professional do to help?

## 12.5.1 Information about cerebral palsy

Cerebral palsy is a condition where the part of the brain controlling movement is damaged. Cerebral palsy is congenital. The brain is abnormal: either it has not developed properly or it was damaged during pregnancy or during birth. There are various types of cerebral palsy:

- quadriplegia: all four limbs are weak
- diplegia or paraplegia: both legs are weak, but not the arms
- hemiplegia: one side of the body is weak
- ataxia: balance is poor and movements unsteady
- dyskinesia: involuntary movements, especially writhing (athetoid) movements, are present.

Many children with cerebral palsy were born prematurely. Sometimes the premature birth occurred because the brain had not developed normally but sometimes part of the brain was damaged during a difficult birth or by a bleed into the brain shortly after birth. The damage to the brain that is responsible for the weakness may cause other problems.

- Low intelligence. Often, but by no means always, present. It is especially likely to occur with diplegia and quadriplegia. Sometimes children with cerebral palsy may be thought to have low intelligence because they have great difficulty making themselves understood. If one helps them to communicate and takes trouble to understand them, it may turn out that they have much higher intelligence than seemed likely. Children with cerebral palsy are often much brighter in some ways than in others.
- Problems with perception. The child may have difficulty telling the difference between shapes, causing delay in learning to read. They may have difficulty finding their way about because they cannot differentiate right from left.
- Coordination of movement. The child may be clumsy either because of weakness or because the part of the brain controlling movement is damaged.
- Feeding problems. The child may have coordination problems with swallowing, making it difficult for them to eat. This means they often put on weight slowly after birth.

Children with cerebral palsy are more likely than other children to have emotional and behaviour problems. They are especially likely to have problems with attention and concentration. The emotional and behaviour problems may occur either because of brain damage or because they face unusual stresses, such as learning difficulties, teasing and humiliation. They may be excluded from activities in which other children take part. This may result in low self-esteem and depression.

The presence of a child with cerebral palsy may cause tensions in the family, with parents disagreeing on how best to manage the child. Brothers and sisters may feel left out. However, there are often positive aspects to having a child with a physical disability in the family. Parents may be drawn closer together, and brothers and sisters may learn that children who are 'different' may still be lovable and make a great contribution to family life.

### 12.5.2 Finding out more about children with cerebral palsy

- Find out the extent of the weakness. What parts of the body are affected and which parts are working well?
- Is the child being given the opportunity to move the weak parts of the body as much as possible? Are the limbs that are very weak being moved regularly so that the joints do not stiffen up?
- How is the child communicating? Can the child's communication be improved?
- Is the child being educated as well as possible? If he has difficulty getting to school, can arrangements be made to help him to get there?
- Is the child being excluded from having friendships with other children? Can more be done to help him to mix with others of his age?
- Does the child have any behaviour or emotional problems? If so, are these receiving attention as suggested in the relevant sections of this book?
- How is the family coping? Can the parents talk to each other about the problems caused by having a child with cerebral palsy? Are other children able to discuss how they feel about having a brother or sister with a disability? What do they see as the positive sides of this situation?
- What do the parents know about the reasons why their child has cerebral palsy? Are they feeling guilty about the disability, thinking they had something to do with causing it?

Now, given the information you have obtained, try to understand how the cerebral palsy is affecting the life of this particular child. Then go on to work out a plan to help.

### 12.5.3 Helping children with cerebral palsy

- Try to develop a good relationship with both the child and the parents so that they trust you.
- Have a discussion with the child about his life, taking into account his ability to communicate.
- After checking weakness and power in the limbs, make sure the weak limbs are being regularly exercised and moved. This will prevent the joints from stiffening up.
- If physiotherapy and/or speech therapy are available locally, make sure that the parents are put in touch with these professionals for further advice. Speech and language therapists may be helpful in providing advice about feeding problems, especially in young children.
- If the child is having problems in school such as learning difficulties, being bullied or difficulties in making friends, contact the school to see whether more help can be provided.
- If the child has an emotional or behaviour problem or difficulties in attention or concentration, make sure that the child and parents are receiving appropriate help (see relevant sections of this book).
- Discuss with the parents their views about the reasons their child has cerebral palsy. Help them to express what may well be inappropriate feelings of guilt.
- Discuss with the parents how they see their child's future. It may be difficult for the parents to make plans for the future, but usually they will appreciate the opportunity to discuss this.

## 12.6 Seizures/fits (epilepsy)

**Case 12.6**

Samir is a 12-year-old boy brought to the clinic by his mother because he has had two seizures. These came on without warning. He had said, 'Mum, I don't feel well' and then a few moments later he fell to the ground with his arms and legs making regular, jerky movements. He did not answer to his name and had noisy breathing. The seizure lasted about 3 minutes, after which Samir gradually seemed to 'wake up'. He got up from the floor and seemed dazed. At this point he had a headache that lasted about an hour. Then he was perfectly all right again. He has not had any fits like this before but when he was a baby he had attacks of shaking when he had a high fever. Nobody else in the family has had seizures. There do not seem to be any unusual stresses in the family. When the health professional examined Samir, he did not have any weakness of his face, arms or legs and he seemed normal. What should the health professional do?

## 12.6.1 Information about seizures/fits

There are two main types of seizure (also referred to as fits or attacks):

1    epileptic seizures
2    non-epileptic seizures.

### Epileptic seizures

In an epileptic seizure there is a sudden discharge of electricity in the brain. This may affect:

- the whole of the brain (generalised seizure), or
- part of the brain (partial seizure).

Reasons for epileptic seizures include:

- family members with epilepsy, particularly febrile convulsions – this suggests a genetic cause;
- pre-existing brain damage or dysfunction – children with developmental problems such as severe intellectual disability, cerebral palsy or autism are more likely to have epilepsy. The brain may have been damaged in the past by a head injury, meningitis or cerebral malaria. Often there is no identifiable condition or illness, occurring in children who have a genetic vulnerability to seizures;
- epileptic attacks that may be triggered by exposure to bright, flashing lights;
- symptomatic seizures that may occur as a result of a brain tumour, an infection in the brain such as meningitis, malaria, tuberculosis, sleeping sickness or tapeworm, or low blood sugar level, especially in a child with diabetes who has taken too much insulin.

In many societies it is believed that a person with fits/seizures is bewitched or is inhabited by evil spirits.

Most children who develop epilepsy need medication on a long-term basis, but they can lead normal lives, go to school and study like other children.

Children with epilepsy have an increased tendency to show behaviour and emotional disorders. These can be caused by the epileptic trigger, by the seizures themselves or by anxiety and the discrimination related to the diagnosis of epilepsy. It may also be caused by normal every day stresses. Most children with epilepsy, however, do not have behaviour or emotional disorders.

### Generalised epileptic seizure

When the whole of the brain is affected (generalised epileptic seizure), the child or adolescent may show some or all of the following signs:

- usually has little warning but may sense that an attack is coming on
- falls to the ground, sometimes after a brief scream or cry
- jerky movements of the arms and legs
- eyeballs may roll upwards
- may go pale or blue because of the lack of oxygen
- is unconscious and does not respond to his name
- may bite his tongue
- may lose control of the bladder and pass urine
- comes round slowly and has a period of confusion or headache, lasting anything from a few minutes to a few hours
- the attack usually lasts a few minutes but may go on for as long as several hours (status epilepticus).

With other types of generalised seizure, the most common indicator is momentary loss of consciousness with staring of the eyes, blinking and, very occasionally, facial twitching. In the classroom, affected children may stop what they are doing, stare vacantly for a brief period and then resume the same activity as before without realising anything has happened. These are called absence attacks or *petit mal* and may occur on their own or alongside generalised epileptic seizures.

### Partial epileptic seizures

Partial seizures present in a variety of ways, depending on where the electrical activity is occurring in the brain. The child is likely to get a warning – an aura – that a seizure is coming. This aura may be a smell or taste, or an unusual sensation often felt in the abdomen. This may be followed by a feeling of fear, tightness of the chest, hallucinations or odd automatic behaviour, such as smacking of the lips. Some partial seizures may cause jerking or weakness of just one part or side of the body (face or limb) and may then sometimes spread to become a more generalised seizure. This can last for a few minutes up to as long as a few hours (partial continuous epilepsy). The child may respond to his name and even carry out requests but is clearly not completely conscious. The attack may be followed by a headache

## Fainting

Another type of attack that may be mistaken for a fit/seizure is a faint. In a faint, a child feels dizzy and unsteady. The child may fall to the floor but will not lose consciousness except perhaps for a moment or so. If the child sits or lies down he immediately begins to feel better. There are usually no jerky movements or other signs of an epileptic seizure. These episodes may follow a temper tantrum or after a sudden surprise. Occasional faints are not a sign of illness and do not require any special treatment. However, children who are ill or dehydrated or hungry are more likely to faint.

## Non-epileptic seizures

Non-epileptic seizures occur both in children who have epileptic seizures and in those without. They are usually brought on by stress. In non-epileptic seizures the child:

- may show a variety of attacks, often different from each other
- may fall to the floor
- may show movements that appear purposeful
- may appear to be unconscious but will often respond to questions or to his name
- will not change colour, pass urine or harm themselves
- will have normal reaction of the pupils to a bright light.

Some infants and young children up to the age of about 4 years have fits/seizures whenever they have a high fever. These fits are called 'febrile convulsions'. When they occur frequently they need the same first aid as for any generalised fit and the child should be undressed and allowed to cool, but not be allowed to get too cold. Paracetamol should be given as soon as possible to reduce the fever. Most children with febrile convulsions do not go on to develop epileptic seizures of the type described above, but a minority do.

## 12.6.2 Finding out more about children with seizures

The first important task when a child or adolescent comes to you with a seizure is to work out what type of seizure it is. You will need to know:

- whether the attack seemed to have been triggered by anything
- exactly what the attack looked like

- what, if any, warning the child had
- whether the child was unconscious, partially conscious or completely conscious during the attack
- how long the attack lasted
- what happened after the attack.

Given this information, you should be able to work out whether the child has had a generalised epileptic seizure, a partial seizure, a non-epileptic seizure or possibly more than one type of attack.

If the child has either a generalised or partial form of epilepsy you will need to decide whether there is a physical cause. Does the child have a temperature or other signs of an infection? Are there signs of meningitis, tuberculosis, sleeping sickness, etc.? A physical examination of the arms and legs to see whether there is any weakness may be helpful. At this point if there is someone with more expertise available, you should refer for further investigation, especially if an underlying illness is suspected or the fits are frequent.

If the child's fits/seizures are apparently non-epileptic and he does not have epileptic seizures, talk to the child and parents about the stresses the child may be experiencing. Remember that generalised or partial fits/seizures may very occasionally also be brought on by stress.

Now, using the information you have obtained from the child with epilepsy or another type of seizure and the family member(s) you have seen, try to understand what has happened and decide what is the best course of action.

### 12.6.3 Helping a child with seizures

The steps below should be followed if you see the child in a fit or are recommending to parents what to do when the child has a fit.

1   Turn the child onto one side.
2   If necessary, remove him from danger and place some soft clothing under his head.
3   Leave the child alone to recover; in particular, do not try to force anything into his mouth, do not try to restrain him and do not force him to take a drink.
4   If the seizure goes on for more than 5 minutes, put a diazepam suppository (0.5 mg/kg) into the child's rectum.
5   If the seizure goes on for more than 10 minutes, insert another diazepam suppository.
6   If the child has an underlying cause for the epilepsy, such at meningitis, tuberculosis, tapeworm or sleeping sickness, then this will need treatment. In the case of meningitis, the need for treatment will be urgent.

A child who has had more than two or three seizures will need medication. Where there is an identifiable underlying cause, treatment will usually be needed for both the underlying cause and the fits if they are recurrent.

#### Medication (anticonvulsants) for fits/seizures

- Medication will reduce or even stop seizures that have been happening repeatedly.
- Some children may need to take medication for the rest of their lives.
- You should use the anticonvulsants recommended on the basis of efficacy and cost.
- Only prescribe one anticonvulsant at a time. That way you will be able to know which medication is causing improvement/side-effects.
- Remember, all anticonvulsants may have side-effects, especially drowsiness and difficulties concentrating, or occasionally behaviour problems such as hyperactivity.

- If the side-effects are severe on the dose of medication needed to stop the fits completely, it may be better to reduce the dose a little and accept that the child may have very occasional fits.

Note that if a child with fits/seizures is showing unusual behaviour between attacks, this may be the result of abnormal brain activity that is not producing a full-blown epileptic attack. It may also be due to an underlying physical or mental health problem. Further investigation including, if possible, an electrocencephalogram should be carried out.

## 12.6.4 Advice to children and parents of children with epilepsy

Children with epilepsy who do not have another disability can lead a normal life, go to school, learn well and later on get a job, marry and have children.

Teenagers with epilepsy should try to lead a healthy lifestyle, drinking alcohol only occasionally, taking part in a normal level of exercise and having regular meals.

Children with epilepsy should not swim unaccompanied because of the very small risk of having a fit in the water and drowning.

## 12.6.5 Community education

Health professionals should take every opportunity to reduce stigma in the community in which they work. Often the most severe disability experienced by a child with epilepsy is not caused by the illness but by the social isolation imposed by other children, other parents and the community. Health professionals should educate the community that epilepsy is not caused by black magic or evil spirits and has nothing to do with supernatural forces. Some parents will not let their children go to school or play with a child with epilepsy because they are worried their children will 'catch' it. Epilepsy is not contagious and cannot be passed on from one child to another like an infection. It is a disorder of the brain.

Now make a list of the ways in which the health professional might be able to help Samir.

# 12.7 Diabetes mellitus

**Case 12.7**

Pranav is a 14-year-old boy brought by his mother to a health clinic on the outskirts of the city. About 6 months ago he was diagnosed with diabetes in a specialised clinic at the main city hospital. He had been referred to the city hospital by the health professional to whom he had now returned. Six months ago he had been suffering from thirst, excessive drinking and loss of weight. His blood and urine had been examined and found to show sugar levels much above normal. At the hospital he had been put on medication and told to lose weight and do more exercise. He had been given a glucometer to measure his blood sugar once a day. At the time he was diagnosed, Pranav was very overweight. Over the past 6 months he had not kept to his diet and had indeed put on weight rather than lost it. He had been taking the medication he had been prescribed but this was expensive, costing about a fifth of the family income. His mother left the use of the glucometer to him but she knew he was not using it regularly. She wanted to go back to the specialist clinic, but the fares to the city hospital were too expensive for more than one person to go and Pranav's mother did not think it was a good idea for Pranav to go by himself. So she had brought him to the health professional who had first made the diagnosis. Pranav had not wanted to come as he thought he would be told off. What can the health professional do?

## 12.7.1 Information about diabetes mellitus

Diabetes mellitus is a disease caused by insulin failure. Insulin is a hormone that regulates blood sugar levels, making sure they do not fall too low or rise too high. There are two types of diabetes:

1   type 1 diabetes – the cells producing insulin are destroyed and so cannot produce insulin. This condition is acute, very serious and if left untreated may result in a coma and then death over a few days or weeks;
2   type 2 diabetes – cells produce insulin but the body does not respond to the hormone, so it is ineffective. This (insulin-resistant) type is closely linked to obesity. It is much more chronic in its course.

Until the 1990s, children and adolescents virtually only had type 1 diabetes. Now, because of the increase in the rate of obesity in many middle-income countries, type 2 diabetes is increasing in frequency.

The increase in the rate of obesity has been caused by teenagers doing less exercise, together with an increase in calorie intake/the amount of food they eat (see Section 6.2).

## 12.7.2 Finding out more about children with diabetes mellitus

The diagnosis of diabetes mellitus is usually fairly easy to make. Excessive thirst, increased urination and loss of weight are the main presenting symptoms in both types, but the course of type 1 diabetes is much more rapid. Patients with either type 1 or type 2 diabets may present with recurrent infections.

It is important to make the diagnosis promptly. Increased thirst may be mistaken as a symptom of anxiety and the diagnosis missed for this reason. A raised sugar level in a simple urine test will make the diagnosis highly probable. Missing a diagnosis of type 1 diabetes can result in a fatal outcome.

Occasionally it is difficult to decide whether an adolescent has type 1 or type 2 diabetes. Most, but not all of those with type 2 diabetes are seriously overweight, while type 1 is not linked to any particular body size. Blood tests are necessary to distinguish between the two.

Assessment should involve judging how well the child and family can cope with the treatment necessary.

Now, given the information you have obtained, try to understand whether the diabetes is being well treated and how it is affecting the life of this particular child. Then go on to work out a plan to help.

## 12.7.3 Helping children with diabetes mellitus

Treatment of both types of diabetes involves first of all education about the condition and its treatment. In type 2 diabets, the importance of increasing exercise and reducing food intake needs to be stressed from the start.

If the child has type 2 diabetes, he will need insulin injections. In type 2 diabetes, oral medication can be tried first, although insulin injection may be required. The child, together with his parents, needs to be taught how to use a glucometer and, if necessary, how to change the amount of insulin or dose of medication accordingly. A specialist nurse or doctor can do this.

There are various ways of delivering insulin. All at the moment require injections either with a needle or an insulin pen.

Inadequately treated diabetes results in the development of many complications. It can reduce vision, affect kidney function and nerves, and lead to ulceration in the legs. The latter is usually seen later on in life in people who have had diabetes for at least 10 years. It is really important that diabetes mellitus is treated as well as possible so that these complications can at least be delayed.

Now, given the information you have obtained, try to understand how this particular child with diabetes is affected in everyday life. Then go on to work out a plan to help.

## 12.7.4 Helping the mental health of children with diabetes mellitus

- Prevention: the health professional should use every opportunity she can to alert parents and children to the dangers of being overweight.
- Practical advice on how to exercise more and how to reduce calorie intake is much more helpful than vague encouragement. Here are some tips.
  - First, ask the teenager what ideas he has for increasing exercise and reducing food intake. Build on these ideas rather than imposing your own ideas, although you may have some new suggestions that the child and family have not thought of.
  - The best exercise is that taken as part of daily life, not as a special activity. Encourage walking or cycling instead of taking a bus to school or when going shopping.
  - Talking to teachers about making regular physical exercise and competitive games a more important part of the curriculum is worthwhile.
  - Avoiding snacking is especially important for weight loss. However, snacking is often an important part of teenage life. Try to help the adolescent to snack on a bottle of water and very low-calorie foods when with friends.
  - Changes in the pattern of exercise and in dietary habits are never easy but are easier if the whole family tries to change at the same time. This is often necessary as if a teenager is overweight, the chances that the parents and siblings are overweight is substantial.
- Keeping in touch with a specialist clinic may be very difficult for a child and family. By using email or telephone, the health professional in a clinic some distance away may be able to help to keep the family in touch with specialist expertise.
- The health professional might put the child and family in touch with other young people with the same condition. A small group of teenagers, some of whom have diabetes and some who are seriously overweight, might be a source of mutual support.
- Non-adherence with treatment is a common problem in teenagers with diabetes mellitus. It may arise from:
  - poor explanation to the teenager about the importance of adherence and the likelihood of complications if the treatment programme is not followed – further explanations may be necessary;
  - a poor relationship between the child and the parents leading to the child using non-adherence as a weapon against his own parents – this will need discussion with both parents and with the child;
  - misery/sadness/depression in the young person leading to low self-esteem and to not caring what happens (see Section 7.7.4);
  - other associated behaviour or emotional problems (see relevant sections for advice).
- Some young people rebel against diabetes and subsequently have a condition that is very difficult to control. These cases need expert, specialist help if at all possible.

Now make a list of the ways in which the health professional might be able to help Pranav.

# 12.8 HIV/AIDS

**Case 12.8**

Shasti is a 9-year-old girl brought to the clinic by her grandmother with whom she lives in a small town in South Africa. Both of Shasti's parents died of AIDS before she was 4 years old. Shasti can hardly remember them because they were too ill to look after her even before they died. Shasti was born HIV negative, but her mother breastfed her and she became HIV positive at about 18 months. She was immediately put on antiretroviral therapy and has been on it ever since. Her outlook is, her grandmother has been told, quite good. She may live well into adult life if she keeps taking the antiretrovirals. However, she is becoming uncooperative. Further, the grandmother is concerned about what will happen when Shasti enters puberty. Girls of 13 and 14 are often sexually active in this part of South Africa. Her grandmother thinks that Shasti does not know that she is HIV positive. At the moment Shasti is a normal, healthy girl. What should she be told? How can the health professional help?

## 12.8.1 Information about psychosocial aspects of HIV/AIDS

Acquired immunodeficiency syndrome (AIDS) is the group of infectious and neurological diseases which people with human immunodeficiency virus (HIV) develop if they are not treated, and from which they die. HIV/AIDS infections are most common in African countries, especially in southern Africa. They do occur nearly everywhere else in the world but much less frequently.

Nearly all HIV infection is passed on during sexual intercourse. It is also transmitted by infected blood during blood transfusion and by infected needles used by drug users. Most children with HIV have been infected in fetal life because the virus was in their mother's bloodstream. A smaller number are infected because the virus was in their mother's breast milk. A very small number are infected as a result of sexual abuse. The false belief that intercourse with a virgin can cure a man with AIDS has led to an additional number of girls being infected.

Untreated, most children with HIV at birth die by the age of 5 years. Treated with antiretroviral therapy, most will survive well into adult life. Although the number of children with HIV treated with antiretroviral therapy has increased, there are still a number of infected children who are not treated. It is really important that children receiving antiretroviral therapy take it regularly if they are to benefit from the treatment. This is often very difficult for carers who are likely to be struggling with a number of other stresses.

HIV infection can be passed on during sexual intercourse even by people who are receiving antiretroviral therapy. People who are on antiretroviral therapy need to use condoms when having intercourse to avoid passing on the infection.

Parents with AIDS often have difficulty looking after their children properly because they are easily tired and may be in pain. If their brain is infected they may become disabled with dementia or other neurological disorders. Children with HIV whose parents die may be resented because they are seen as a burden. Many children with HIV infection are orphaned in early life, are looked after by relatives or in institutions, or live in child-headed households.

Children with HIV for whom treatment is not available show:

- feeding problems
- failure to thrive
- repeated infections
- slow speech development
- if the child survives long enough, gradual deterioration of intelligence
- increased rates of behaviour and emotional problems.

Children with HIV are often discriminated against even in parts of the world where the disease is common. Parents and grandparents may feel guilt and shame about the condition. Many children with HIV infection have not been told of their diagnosis to protect them from painful news about their parents and themselves. This puts those with whom they have intercourse later in life at considerable risk of developing the infection.

Families with a child with HIV are likely to be living in poverty.

In many places where HIV is prevalent there are clinics available to counsel children, adolescents and adults with this condition. Pregnant women are in particular need of counselling. These clinics also counsel carers who are looking after children whose parents have died from HIV.

## 12.8.2 Finding out more about children with HIV/AIDS

- Find out about the social circumstances in which the child is living. Is the child living with the parents or were they unable to look after the child? Who is living with and looking after the child?
- Is the child being well looked after or is he being neglected because his presence is resented as an additional burden, or because there are no adults looking after him?
- Is the child receiving antiretroviral therapy? If not, can this be obtained? If the child is receiving it, is it being taken regularly? It is worth asking the child why he is taking this medicine.
- If the child is not receiving antiretroviral therapy regularly, why is this? Is the child being resistant, are the carers being negligent in this respect or are there difficulties in obtaining the medication?
- What has the child been told? Does the child know about his condition and its implications for later life? If not, why has the child not been told?
- Does the child have any behaviour or emotional problems?
- Is the child attending school regularly? If not, is this because the carers have unrealistic ideas about other children at school catching the disease? Or is it because they are ashamed and do not want the family to be humiliated? Or is it because they cannot afford the school fees?
- In the case of a teenage girl, is she sexually active? If so, is she using contraception?
- Has the family been put in touch with the local HIV counselling service?

Now, using the information you have obtained from the child with HIV/AIDS and the family member(s) you have seen, try to understand what has happened and decide what is best to do.

## 12.8.3 Helping children with HIV/AIDS

- Discuss the care of the child with whoever is looking after him. Note any problems arising from shame and guilt over the cause of the child's condition. Make sure the carers (parents or others who have taken over the parental role) realise you are sympathetic to them and understand how they feel. Make it clear that you do not blame them for anything that has happened. It is just your job to help as much as you can.
- If the child is receiving antiretroviral therapy, check that this is being taken regularly. If there are problems with adherence, then take steps as suggested in Chapter 17. Note that it may be very hard for carers to ensure adherence if they have other stresses to cope with. If the child is not receiving antiretroviral therapy, find out whether this can be made available to him.
- Identify any problems in development the child may have and offer advice on how to promote development (see Section 15.4).

- If the child is not attending school regularly, find out why this is and see whether you can offer advice to improve school attendance.
- In the case of a sexually active teenage girl not using contraception, make sure the girl is given and has access to contraceptive advice.
- Identify any behaviour or emotional problems the child may have and offer management along the lines suggested in the relevant sections elsewhere in this manual.
- Help the carers to discuss the child's HIV status with the child as well as its implications for later life. Put the carers in touch with the local HIV counselling service if there is one.

Now make a list of the ways in which the health professional might be able to help Shasti.

# 12.9 Sickle cell disease

**Case 12.9**

Nelson is a 9-year-old boy with known sickle cell disease who was brought to the health clinic with acute pain in his legs and shoulders. He was crying with the pain which he had had many times before. The health professional gave him some tablets for pain relief and then enquired about his life at home and school. It turned out that he was missing a great deal of school, sometimes because of the painful episodes but often because his mother kept him at home just in case he had another attack. What should the health professional do?

## 12.9.1 Information about sickle cell disease

This is a disorder of the blood caused by a defect in haemoglobin. The defect causes the red blood cells to clump together and block small blood vessels. This results in a reduction of oxygen supply to the tissue, producing acute pain lasting a few hours to several days. Episodes of pain can be triggered by infection, cold or dehydration, but sometimes there is no obvious trigger. The frequency of pain is very variable. The condition is an autosomal recessive genetic blood disorder. Both parents are carriers of the gene but are unaffected. If both parents are carriers, there is a one in four risk of their having a child with sickle cell disease. The child may have anaemia and require occasional blood transfusions. The condition occurs all over the world but mostly in sub-Saharan Africa.

If it is possible for children to take folic acid as a supplement and penicillin from 3 months of age this will prevent pneumococcal infection to which children with sickle cell disease are prone. This needs to be taken for at least the first 5 years, but preferably on a lifelong basis. Children need to be well hydrated, especially when in hot environments or when exercising.

Treatment of the condition mainly consists of managing the painful episodes with analgesics such as paracetamol and anti-inflammatory agents; sometimes opioids will be needed. The child should also be given fluids by mouth.

The painful episodes affect both family and school life, with numerous school absences. Affected children should be encouraged to take a full part in school life. They may be anxious between episodes about when the next attack will occur. With good medical management, children with this condition can survive into late adulthood.

Parents should bring a child with this condition back to the health professional if the child runs a high fever, becomes very pale or develops breathing difficulties.

## 12.9.2 Finding out about children with sickle cell disease

The diagnosis requires laboratory facilities which are available in places where the condition is endemic. Blood samples should be sent away if the condition is suspected and there are no such facilities available locally.

- Does the child have anaemia? If so, he may need a blood transfusion.
- Is the child receiving appropriate pain management when painful episodes occur? Most pain can be managed at home.
- Does the child have any behaviour or emotional problems? In particular, is he so anxious between attacks that his ability to attend school is affected?
- What is the attitude of the parent(s)? Do they ensure that the child gets appropriate pain management? Are they so anxious between attacks that they are unnecessarily preventing the child from leading as normal a life as possible?
- Do the teachers know about the child's medical problem? Are they well informed about what to do when the child has a painful crisis?

Now, using the information you have obtained from the child with sickle cell disease and the family member(s) you have seen, try to understand how the condition is being managed and decide what the best course of action is.

### 12.9.3 Helping children with sickle cell disease

In most areas where sickle cell disease is widespread there is a community-based pain management service available. This service will also be able to carry out blood tests, check whether the child has anaemia and perform blood transfusions if necessary.

The health professional responsible needs to be familiar with the best means of pain management, using analgesics and how to manage other common complications such as infection, pain arising from the spleen and acute chest conditions.

If the assessment has revealed that the child's life is more limited than really needs to be the case, the health professional needs to see the parents and child both together and separately to counsel them on how the child can be helped to lead a more normal life. The health professional should make contact with the child's teachers to ensure they are also involved in helping the child to lead as normal a life as possible.

The genetics of the condition need to be discussed with the parents (and eventually with the child) to make sure that they are aware of the risks of having another child with the condition. If appropriate, they should be given effective contraceptive advice.

As the child gets older, he will need to be able to discuss his condition so that he can gradually take over responsibility for his own healthcare.

Now describe what the health professional might be able to do to help Nelson.

## 12.10 Mental health aspects of life-threatening illness

**Case 12.10**

Manasa is a 10-year-old girl brought to the health professional in a clinic in a poor rural area by her mother, with weakness, breathlessness, severe loss of weight and loss of appetite. She has had a chronic cough and breathlessness for the past 2 years. A diagnosis of tuberculosis was made a year ago and Manasa was put on anti-tuberculosis drugs. These had only been taken irregularly and her condition had gradually worsened. It was now clear that Manasa was terminally ill. It had already been explained to the parents that this was a chronic illness, and that if she did not take the tablets, Manasa would die before she reached adult life. Now her chest condition seems worse and her mother had noticed she has lost a great deal of weight. The health professional, from her previous experience, thinks that Manasa probably only has a few weeks to live. Both Manasa and her mother look very anxious. What should the health professional do?

## 12.10.1 Information about life-threatening illness

In poor areas of LAMI countries, most deaths in childhood are caused by a combination of malnutrition and infectious disease and occur in the first 2–3 years of life, although it is also common later in childhood.

The five most common causes of childhood deaths are pneumonia, diarrhoeal diseases, malaria, measles and malnutrition, the last being an underlying cause in more than half the deaths. Tuberculosis is also a very common cause of death and AIDS is another significant cause in many parts of southern Africa. In infants, birth asphyxia is a common cause of death.

In contrast, in high-income countries and in areas of LAMI countries where nutrition is adequate, most childhood deaths occur in the first year of life from genetic disorders such as congenital heart disease and other congenital malformations. In later childhood and adolescence, most life-threatening illness in high-income countries and affluent areas of LAMI countries arises from cancer, cystic fibrosis and congenital malformations. The most common cancer is acute lymphoblastic leukaemia, for which highly specialist, expensive treatments are effective.

Mental health problems in life-threatening illnesses are similar to those in chronic illnesses that are not life-threatening (see Section 12.1.2), but there are additional issues. These will be summarised here.

When children and adolescents enter the terminal phase of an illness, health professionals such as doctors and nurses often see their main role as prolonging life. This is the case even when it is clear that the quality of life will be very poor. Many health professionals find it difficult to accept that perhaps a more important task is to help make the last few weeks/months as comfortable and meaningful to the child and family as possible. The presence of a life-threatening illness will always have a marked impact on the lives of parents and of the child.

Nearly all families in LAMI countries with a child with a terminal illness will view the illness as having religious meaning. They are likely to visit their temple, mosque or church asking for divine intervention. When the child dies, they will continue to belive that the child's spirit lives on, for which they are likely to pray and consult with their local priests.

As with other chronic illnesses, a life-threatening disorder may put stress on the parents' relationship, resulting in arguments and quarrels. Such a stress may, however, also bring parents closer together as they face a common threat.

A terminal illness may add financial burdens to the family budget, perhaps because of the need for medication or travelling to hospital appointments. Such expenditure on one child may make other children in the family resentful. The lives of brothers and sisters of the child with a chronic illness will, of course, often be affected in other ways.

Parents usually wish to protect their children against the knowledge of the fatal nature of their illness. However, most children are aware of the seriousness of their condition, although many do not talk about it because they wish to protect their parents from distress.

## 12.10.2 Finding out more about the child with a chronic life-threatening illness

- If at all possible, some time should be spent alone with the parent(s) and some time alone with the child.
- Make sure that, as far as resources permit, the child's illness is being treated appropriately, especially as far as relief of distressing symptoms, such as pain and breathlessness, are concerned.
- Find out whether the parents have a realistic idea of the length of life that can be expected. Check how much they think the child knows about the likely outcome.
- If there are genetic implications of the child's condition, are the parents aware of these?

For example, parents with a child with sickle cell disease have a one in four chance of having another child with the same disorder.

- Ask about the effect the illness is having on the child's life as well as on the lives of other members of the family.
- Ask about the religious practices that the family observes.
- Ask about any financial implications of the illness and whether the family can manage on their resources.
- If the child is still at school, check whether he is having any difficulties getting there. Is the child being bullied at school? Are the teachers well informed about the nature of the child's illness?
- Are the parents being appropriately protective of the child? Is the child being allowed to do as much as one might reasonably expect given the nature of his illness? Is he being overprotected? Is he being rejected and very much left to fend for himself?

### 12.10.3 Promoting the mental health of children with chronic life-threatening illness

Ensure the parents are well informed of the genetic implications of their child's condition and that he is being treated appropriately with the best available symptom management. Be aware that it is desirable to use sufficient medication to relieve symptoms even if the medication might shorten life.

Encourage communication about the illness within the family and between the parents and the school. If at all possible, see both parents together so that any disagreements between them can be discussed.

Health professionals are likely to share the same beliefs of their patients concerning the religious meaning of the terminal illness of a child and the afterlife. If the health professional is from a different culture and does not share the same beliefs, she should not discourage these beliefs as they are usually a source of great comfort. In addition, she should encourage the family to use all the community supports available. Close family and friends, priests or ministers of religion and traditional healers may all provide such support.

If appropriate, arrange to see the parents after the child has died to enable them to express their feelings about what has happened. Encourage them to talk with their other children about what has happened, so that the child who has died can be talked about in the family without anxiety or embarrassment.

Now make a list of the ways in which the health professional might be able to help Manasa.

CHAPTER 13

# Physical illness without an identifiable physical explanation

Virtually every symptom that can be the result of a physical illness may also arise from a non-physical cause. Lack of energy, stomach aches, headaches, pains anywhere in the body, inability to walk or to talk, and difficulties with hearing/sight may all occur for non-physical reasons but be equally as disabling as if a physical illness were present.

## 13.1 Assessment of physical symptoms

As a health professional your main task will be to assess, diagnose and provide treatment for the physical conditions for which patients attend the clinic. However, research has shown that for a number of patients who come to clinics with physical symptoms (perhaps one in four or one in five), it is not possible to make a medical diagnosis. This is true for children as well as adults. These children need your help just as much as those for whom a physical diagnosis can be made.

In this chapter we provide a general account of ways you can be helpful for the children who fall into this group. Many health professionals find patients for whom a physical diagnosis cannot be made very irritating. They may even get frustrated and angry with these patients. But if you become interested in this type of problem, you will find dealing with it just as rewarding as the rest of your work. How to assess the problem will depend on the main problem the parent talks about.

### 13.1.1 Assessing a physical symptom or symptoms

Your first task is to find out whether the child has a physical illness or disorder. In a number of children that you see, it is either not possible to make a diagnosis of a physical illness at all or a physical problem is present but cannot account for the degree of disability that the child is exhibiting. This chapter aims to help you to deal with these common situations.

> **Case 13.1**
> A 7-year-old boy, Ali, is brought to you with moderately severe abdominal pain. He is not going to school or playing with his friends. He is eating normally. There is no vomiting or diarrhoea. When you examine the boy you find he looks well, is growing normally, has no temperature, has a normal pulse rate and when you press on the abdomen, there is no localised tenderness or rebound tenderness. The urine is normal. You decide that there is almost certainly no physical illness present.

How do you proceed to find out more? There are various principles to bear in mind when deciding what to do next.

You need to know what the parent thinks the pain is caused by. Are they absolutely convinced that there is something physically wrong with their son? Perhaps another child they know has had a serious illness and they are worried that their child has the same problem. Or do they already suspect the problem is not physical but has something to do with the way their son is reacting to stress? Or do they really have no idea what is going on? All three are quite possible. So you need to ask, for example, 'Why do you think your son has the pain?' and 'What do you think is causing it?'

You need to communicate that you understand there is obviously something wrong but that it is not a physical illness. In doing this you need to make clear that although it is good news that the child does not have a physical illness, you need to try to work out why he has the pain. It is important that you do not convey that because he does not have a physical illness, there is really nothing wrong with him. Clearly, if he cannot go to school or play with his friends there is something really very wrong. So you need to say something such as 'I'm pretty sure that Ali does not have a physical illness. But of course there is something wrong here. We must try to find out what it is. Do you have any ideas?'

Explore a range of stress possibilities. At this point, if you have time, it would be a good idea with children over the age of 8 years to see them separately. If you are not seeing children separately, make sure you include the child in discussions with the parent about possible stresses. You can ask questions such as 'I wonder whether there is anything at school that is upsetting him? What do you think about that, [name of child]?' and 'Or anything at home? What about that, [name of child]?'

While you are talking with the parent, do note how the child reacts, especially during discussion about stresses. Children will sometimes make clear that they do or do not agree with what their parent is saying. Occasionally, they will say what they think, but even if they do not, the expression on their face may tell you a great deal.

Shame, guilt, fear and loyalty may all stop parents talking freely about stresses in the home. A mother may be ashamed of her husband's drink problem, guilty about having hit her child, frightened of what her husband will do to her if she talks about his jealousy, or feel too loyal to her husband to want to talk about what she sees as some of his failings as a father. You need to show that you are aware of how hard it is to talk about stresses by saying things such as 'I know it may be very hard to talk about some of these things' and 'Maybe there are things you do not want to talk about, but perhaps you could just say whether you know what is upsetting him even if you do not want to say what it is?'

Be sensitive about asking questions the parent may not like being asked. When asking questions about stresses you may feel that you are being too personal or intrusive. You need to acknowledge when you think this might be the case, for example: 'I'm sorry. I think it's very hard for you to think about this. Maybe you would prefer not to talk about it?' Remember though that it may be necessary for the parent to feel some emotional distress if they are to help their child. Causing emotional upset is not something a health professional likes doing, but just as it may be necessary to cause pain when diagnosing abdominal pain arising from appendicitis, so too might it be necessary to probe painful topics when finding out what is upsetting a child.

After 10–15 minutes you will probably be in one of the following situations.

- You have a fairly good idea of why the child has disabling physical symptoms without a physical illness being present. Further, you may be able to offer some advice about what to do to reduce or even eliminate the stress. For example, the child may be being bullied at school and you might suggest to the parent the importance of discussing this with the child's teacher.

- You may have identified the probable stress, but not be able to think of anything that will help to reduce or eliminate it. In this situation you will be able to suggest ways of achieving symptomatic relief (see Section 13.3.3).
- You may have very little or no idea what is upsetting the child. Again, you will be able to suggest ways of achieving symptomatic relief (see Section 13.3.3).

Aims you should hope to have achieved by the end of an assessment include the following:

- you should have ruled out physical illness with a considerable degree of certainty
- the parent should at least be in the position of considering the possibility that their child's symptoms do not have a physical cause
- you should have explored possible stresses causing the pain
- you and the parent should both have a plan of what to do next
- the parent and child should both feel encouraged and supported by you rather than humiliated by the knowledge that the child does not have a physical illness.

## 13.2 Weakness without physical cause

**Case 13.2**

Gethera is a 13-year-old girl carried into the clinic by her parents because she cannot walk. They said that their daughter stopped walking about a week ago. About 10 days before, she had a flu-like illness, with a temperature, shivering and cough. This cleared up and she seemed a lot better. But then one morning, when it seemed she was nearly ready to return to school, she called her parents and told them that she could not move her legs. They were naturally very alarmed and wanted to take her to the clinic straight away, but she said she did not want to go to the clinic. Her legs would get better and she was frightened of the clinic. So they did not take her but brought her meals in bed and helped her to go to the toilet by half carrying her there. But after a week they decided they would have to come to the clinic whether Gethera wanted to go or not. When they came in, Gethera was crying, saying she did not want to see the health professional. Her parents put her in a chair and the health professional noticed immediately that she moved her legs to get them into a more comfortable position. When the health professional examined her she found that when she lifted Gethera's legs and then let go, Gethera gradually lowered her legs, showing that she did have power in them. The reflexes in her legs were normal. The health professional asked the parents what they thought and they said that they suspected Gethera could move her legs. Indeed, they thought that sometimes she got up in the night without telling them, to go to the toilet. What should the health professional do?

### 13.2.1 Information about physical symptoms without an identifiable physical explanation (conversion disorder)

The physical symptoms most commonly involve inability to walk, a limp, weakness of an arm or hand, deafness, blindness or milder hearing or visual problems. The condition is sometimes called hysterical paralysis or conversion disorder. Symptoms may arise because the child is under stress or occur following a viral infection or other illness. However, they may also arise for no obvious reason. It may be hard for the parents or child to admit that there is a mental health problem. A physical symptom is a more acceptable way of asking for help from a health professional.

The health professional needs to recognise the wish for help, but to be astute enough to realise that there is no physical problem present. The sooner the health professional realises that there is no physical problem, the quicker the child's real problems can be dealt with. The temptation to carry out a large number of investigations should be avoided. If there are important investigations needed to exclude serious illnesses, these should be done early on together, not one by one. The diagnosis is made first by exclusion of physical illness and then by the fact that the problem is not consistently present. For example, a child who appears unable to walk may be able to show muscular power in the legs in some circumstances but not in others. There may be an underlying depressive condition or, very occasionally, a psychosis.

There may be a tendency in the family to experience physical complaints for which there does not seem to be a physical explanation.

The child's attitude to his disability may be one of distress or of surprising lack of concern.

## 13.2.2 Finding out more about a child with physical symptoms without an identifiable physical cause

- Take a careful history:
  - When did the problem begin?
  - Was the onset sudden or gradual?
  - Was it accompanied by any other symptoms such as fever or headache?
  - Were any other parts of the body affected?
  - Is the symptom consistent or is it variable?
  - Has such an episode occurred before?
  - Has the child had any fits/seizures?
  - Is the child under stress at home, at school, in the neighbourhood?
  - Has anyone in the family or at school had a similar problem?
- Carry out an examination by first asking the child what the problem is.
- Ask the child about his life and listen carefully to what he says.
- Ask whether there are any difficult things happening at home or at school at the present time?
- Carry out as full an examination as you can. For example, if the child is unable to walk, examine especially the legs for power and reflexes, noting whether the signs are consistent with any known neurological disorder.
- Observe whether there is any variation in the symptom. If the symptom is present at some times but not others, it is more likely that the problem is not physical.
- Note whether the child seems upset by the problem or seems untroubled by it.
- If after you have taken a history and carried out an examination you have made a physical diagnosis, then you need to treat the physical condition.
- If, however, you are uncertain whether the child has a physical condition or you are sure the child does not have such a disorder, then, if possible, refer to a more experienced clinician. If there is no one more experienced to whom you can refer, then treat as if the condition is not physical. Keep an open mind and reconsider if new symptoms occur.

Now, using the information you have obtained from the child with such physical symptoms without an obvious physical cause and the family member(s) you have seen, try to understand what has happened and decide what is the best course of action.

## 13.2.3 Helping a child with physical symptoms without an obvious physical cause

- Explain to the child and parents that you have not been able to find a physical explanation for the problem.

- Make clear that this does not mean there is nothing wrong. Obviously there is something wrong or the child would not have the symptom.
- Ask the child and family whether they can explain why the problem has occurred – sometimes such symptoms appear because a child is upset about something.
- If the child is under stress, work out with the family how this can be reduced.
- In any case, tell the child and family that you expect the symptom to gradually improve but that it can get better more quickly with treatment.
- With the child and family devise a programme of very gradual rehabilitation. If you have someone to work with in rehabilitation, all the better.
- With the child, set targets for a gradual recovery, one day at a time.
- At the same time, continue to give the child opportunities to talk about what is worrying him. Occasionally, for example, a history of abuse emerges during rehabilitation.
- Note you should always keep under review the possibility that the child has a physical problem, especially if new physical symptoms or signs emerge. Remember too that sometimes new physical symptoms may be caused by things that are still causing the child upset or stress.

Now make a list of the ways in which the health professional might be able to help Gethera.

## 13.3 Stomach aches

**Case 13.3**

Jamil is a 10-year-old boy brought by his mother to the health clinic with abdominal pains, present for several months. The pains are often quite severe and he sometimes curls up in pain. He also sometimes has pains in other parts of his body, especially his legs. The pains are episodic and last for a few hours at most. He has vomited once or twice with the pain. He has no other symptoms, no diarrhoea or constipation. He is doing reasonably well at school, although his mother says he does not like going very much. At the time he was brought to the clinic he was in the middle of an attack. He looked tense and unhappy. On examining him, he did not have a temperature. When he was asked to point to where the pain was he pointed to all over his abdomen. When his abdomen was pressed he did not show any signs of distress. There was no localised tenderness even with deep palpation and no rebound tenderness when the health professional suddenly removed her hand from the abdomen. His urine was normal. Having failed to find a physical cause for the pain, the health professional asked more detailed questions about when the pain occurred. It turned out that the pain almost always began on Sunday evenings and was often at its worst on Monday mornings when he was sometimes allowed to stay at home because of the pain. The pain virtually never occurred during the school holidays.

## 13.3.1 Information about recurrent, non-organic abdominal pain

In high-income countries, non-organic abdominal pain is far more common than abdominal pain caused by physical disease. This is not the case in LAMI countries, but non-organic pain does occur in these countries too.

Non-organic abdominal pain occurs equally frequently in boys and girls. It is linked to depression and anxiety in both the child and parents, and to non-organic pain elsewhere in the body, especially headache. It sometimes occurs before a stressful experience such as going to school, but more often there is no such obvious link.

## 13.3.2 Finding out more about a child with stomach aches

The health professional should take a careful account of the pain from the parent and child.

- When did it start?
- How long does it last when it occurs?
- Are there other gastrointestinal symptoms: diarrhoea, constipation, blood in the stools, vomiting?
- What is the child's appetite like?
- Has the child lost weight?
- What is the child's general health like? Are there any other physical symptoms?
- Does the pain stop the child from everyday activities, going to school, playing with his friends?
- Is the timing of the pain associated with stress?

The health professional should also carry out a physical examination.

- Weigh the child
- Take the child's temperature
- Examine the child's abdomen, palpating for tenderness and rebound tenderness
- Look for other signs of physical illness
- Examine a specimen of urine
- Carry out an abdominal X-ray if indicated and if facilities are available.

If no organic cause for the child's pain (e.g. appendicitis, infestation, giardisis, abdominal tuberculosis, urinary tract lesions, amoebic colitis) is found, consider the possibility of non-organic pain. Differences between organic and non-organic pain are shown in Table 13.1.

Table 13.1 Organic *v.* non-organic pain

|  | Organic pain | Non-organic pain |
| --- | --- | --- |
| Type of pain | Localised | Diffuse |
| Pain elsewhere in body | Unusual | Common |
| Pain wakes child at night | Often | Rarely |
| Vomiting | May be present | May be present |
| Emotional state | Usually normal | Usually tense, anxious |
| Abnormalities on examination and investigation | Present | Absent |
| Timing related to stress | Unusual | More frequent |

Now, using the information you have obtained from the child with the stomach ache and the family member(s) you have seen, try to understand what has happened and decide what is the best course of action.

### 13.3.3 Helping children with non-organic stomach aches

Explain to the parent and child that no serious physical disorder is present but clearly something is wrong. What does the parent think the pain might be due to? Explain the following possibilities:

- the pain is part of a general emotional upset
- there is no general upset, but the child's pain is due to stress that may or may not be obvious
- there is no clear stress or emotional disturbance, but the child may be reacting to stresses that are not obvious.

If the child's pain appears to be part of a general emotional disturbance, most likely an anxiety state, then if the parent accepts this possibility, follow the guidelines on the management of anxiety (see the relevant sections on helping anxiety in Chapter 7).

If there is no general disturbance and time allows, explore what stressful circumstances may be important here (see the relevant sections on helping anxiety in Chapter 7). Act to remove or reduce stress if at all possible. If the expertise is available, a course of relaxation or CBT be helpful (see Section 2.3.1).

If it remains unclear whether the problem is organic or non-organic, then explain that the pain is likely to clear up over the next few days or weeks. Paracetamol may be useful symptomatically.

Reassure the parents and child that the presence of serious organic illness is extremely unlikely, but add that the pain may recur, in which case the child will need to be seen again (remember that children with non-organic abdominal pain may develop organic disease in the future).

Now make a list of the ways in which the health professional might be able to help Jamil.

## 13.4 Headaches

**Case 13.4**

Tara is a 9-year-old girl who came to the health clinic with her mother, who said that Tara had been complaining of headaches for several weeks. The headaches occurred in her forehead and occasionally on top of her head. They had been present for about 6 weeks. They seemed to occur in the mornings and evenings when she was at home and not at school. They never woke her at night. Tara said the pain is 'like a pressure'. It was continuous and not throbbing. It was partly but not completely relieved by paracetamol. Tara was doing well at school, where she had friends. She was a rather tense girl who easily got upset if things did not go well for her. There did not seem to be any particular stresses at home. Her mother said that she and her husband got on well together. There was an older sister and a younger brother who did not have any problems. What can the health professional do to help?

### 13.4.1 Information about headaches

There are three types of headache:

1   organic headaches: these have a physical cause (unusual)

2   migraine headaches: relatively common
3   non-organic headaches (tension headache): very common.

## Organic headaches

Organic headaches may be caused by:

- short-sightedness, needing spectacles
- infection of the teeth or sinuses
- brain tumours or other brain disease such as cerebral abscess
- brain infections such as meningitis
- diseases of the blood vessels such as aneurysms, stroke or high blood pressure
- epilepsy
- other rare diseases.

Organic headaches are often continuous, worse in the evening and may interfere with sleep.

## Migraine headaches

Migraine headaches do not usually start until 8 or 9 years old. A migraine attack:

- often begins with blurry vision in one eye, a blind spot, and a sensation of vague, dancing shapes in front of the eye
- may be all that is experienced, but may be followed by:
  - a throbbing headache on one side of the head
  - nausea and vomiting
  - avoidance of the light (photophobia)
- varies in the side of the head that is affected; if it always occurs on the same side, an organic cause is more likely
- usually lasts less than half an hour but may go on for hours
- may be triggered by:
  - eating various foods or food additives such as chocolate, nuts, cheese or glutamates
  - stress or the removal of stress
  - strenuous physical exercise
  - a mixture of the above
- is caused by the narrowing and then expanding of small arteries, putting pressure on pain receptors
- may delay sleep, but does not wake the person up
- may be followed by drowsiness or sleep
- may be shortened by paracetamol or anti-migraine medication, especially if taken early in the attack.

## Non-organic headaches

Non-organic headaches are sometimes called tension headaches, but it is often impossible to identify any stress that is causing them. They:

- usually occur daily
- are usually in the front of the head but may feel like tightness, pressure or a 'band' around the head; there may be mild throbbing
- often run in families
- may occur at times of tension, such as before school or a party
- may be accompanied by anxiety or depression
- may overlap in symptoms with migraine headaches

- may be helped by a mild painkiller such as paracetamol
- may occur when the child gets some benefit from them such as being allowed to avoid school or a teacher he does not like.

There is significant overlap between migraine and non-organic headaches.

### 13.4.2 Finding out more about children with headaches

Listen to the account given by the parent and child, and ask questions such as:

- When did the headaches begin?
- Where do they occur and what do they feel like to the child – throbbing, continuous?
- Do they start with 'odd' sensations in front of one eye and/or with a 'blind spot'?
- What part of the day are they worst?
- Do they wake the child at night?
- What seems to trigger them or set them off: certain foods, stress or relief from stress, position the head is held?
- Are there any stresses in the family or at school?
- Is the child getting any benefit from the headaches?
- Does the child have difficulty reading?
- Is there any weakness of the arms or legs?
- Does the child have toothache?
- Has the child had any fits?

The child will then need a brief physical examination.

- Does the child have a temperature?
- Take the blood pressure.
- Check eyesight for short-sightedness.
- Check the mouth and teeth.

A brief physical examination should reveal any weakness of the arms or legs suggestive of a brain disease.

A skull X-ray and a magnetic resonance imaging scan will only be required in the unusual situation when the account or examination suggests an organic cause affecting the brain.

Now, using the information you have obtained from the child or adolescent with headaches and the family member(s) you have seen, try to understand what has happened and decide what is the best course of action.

### 13.4.3 Helping children with headaches

This will depend on what type of headache the health professional thinks the child has after listening to the parents and child, and carrying out an examination. If the headache is thought to be organic, the health professional will need to continue his investigations, then treat or refer on for treatment of the underlying cause. Remember that some organic causes of headache are medical emergencies and require rapid intervention; for example, severe headache with a temperature and stiff neck is likely to be caused by meningitis.

For migraine headaches, first try and eliminate or reduce possible triggers, including foods (especially chocolate and cheese) and additives (especially glutamates). The removal or reduction of stressful triggers will require more detailed enquiries, followed by, for example, trying to change what is going on in school. Treat migraine headaches with medication, paracetamol or anti-migraine tablets.

Non-organic (tension) headaches need management along similar lines to migraine headaches. If stresses can be identified, take steps to reduce or eliminate them. If the child is gaining some benefit, such as being allowed to be absent from school, then work out ways in which the benefit is reduced, for example not being allowed to watch television if the child is off school.

In a number of children it is not possible to identify a cause (e.g. stress for headaches), yet the symptom may persist. In these cases the health professional should explain that the headache almost certainly is not caused by anything serious and that it will probably disappear with time. If the pain is disabling, then muscle relaxation techniques (see p. 53) may be helpful. If psychological expertise is available, a course of CBT is sometimes effective (see Section 2.3.1). Paracetamol or anti-migraine medication may be indicated if the headache is severe and persistent.

Now make a list of the ways in which the health professional might be able to help Tara.

# 13.5 Tiredness/fatigue

### Case 13.5
Fourteen-year-old Anand was brought by his father to the clinic. Anand's father said that for the past 6 months his son was always tired and lacking in energy. He did not seem to be able to get up in the morning and when his father insisted he got up, he took ages to dress and was always late for school. In the afternoon when he came home he did not want to do the homework he was given and just sat in front of the television. Occasionally he would go out, came back home late and was even more tired the next morning. Anand did not seem worried about his lack of energy, but he did complain of numerous physical symptoms, especially headache, ringing in his ears and tingling in his hands. He has had difficulty getting off to sleep, wakes two or three times in the night, and does not want to get up in the morning. He does not seem able to concentrate on his schoolwork. Before this trouble began he was an energetic boy who liked to see his friends, but now he has no interest in his friends. He had been a good student, but now he is failing in school. What should the health professional do?

## 13.5.1 Information about lack of energy

Lack of energy can have a number of causes, both physical and psychological or both. Physical causes include:

- anaemia
- chronic infections, including tuberculosis, HIV, sleeping sickness and malaria
- infestations
- malnutrition
- chronic physical illness
- a combination of the above, with perhaps a chronic infection resulting in lack of appetite, causing malnutrition and anaemia.

Non-physical (psychological) causes include:

- depression
- anxiety
- psychosis
- physical symptoms without a physical cause

- excessive drug (especially marijuana) or alcohol use
- a combination of the above.

## 13.5.2 Assessment of lack of energy

It is first important to find out whether there is a physical problem. You will need to ask about:

- symptoms suggestive of fever, sweats, diarrhoea, blood in urine or faeces
- adequate diet
- any other physical symptoms.

You will then need to take the child's temperature and carry out a full physical examination to see whether he:

- looks malnourished, has dry skin, is underweight
- has any signs of chronic physical illness, such as pallor, difficulty breathing or jaundice.

Then examine a specimen of urine for evidence of infection and a specimen of faeces for signs of infestation.

If there is no physical problem accounting for the lack of energy, then you should try to work out the nature of the psychological problem. This might be:

- depression – as well as lack of energy, does the child show:
  - generally low mood, sadness, unhappiness
  - difficulties sleeping
  - lack of interest in everyday activities he normally enjoys
  - difficulties in attention and concentration
  - ideas of self-harming
- anxiety symptoms, such as fearfulness and excessive worrying.

In some areas, older adolescents and young men show a pattern of tiredness, difficulties sleeping, physical symptoms, irritability and difficulties in concentration and attention known as brain fag syndrome. This syndrome is probably a local expression of a depressive problem.

Drugs, especially marijuana or cannabis (use local terminology) use, may be another reason. As well as asking the teenager about cannabis use, you can ask the parents whether they have noticed the characteristic smell. In addition, ask the teenager about the presence of hallucinations ('Do you sometimes hear voices or sounds?') and delusions ('Do you get the feeling you are being watched, or that people are against you?', 'Does anything strange or odd seem to be happening to you?', 'Do you get the idea that people are interfering with your thoughts?').

In Western society, lack of energy is often regarded as part of normal adolescence. But it is unwise to regard lack of energy as part of normal adolescence unless physical and psychological reasons have been ruled out. Note especially that it is dangerous to regard lack of energy as normal if it is accompanied by ideas of self-harm.

Now, using the information you have obtained from the young person with lack of energy and the family member(s) you have seen, try to understand what has happened and decide what is the best course of action.

## 13.5.3 Helping children who lack energy

This will depend entirely on the results of the assessment, as described earlier. If there is physical illness present, this will need treatment. If there is no physical illness present, most commonly lack of energy is part of a depressive state. For management of this problem, see Section 7.7.4.

Now make a list of the ways in which the health professional might be able to help Anand.

# CHAPTER 14

# Stressful situations

## 14.1 Parental marriage relationships and children

**Case 14.1**

Odra, a 7-year-old girl, was brought to the clinic by her mother with a number of problems that had been going on for several months. These included bed-wetting, fears of going to school (although she had previously liked school), and not wanting to play with her friends. Her mother said that these problems had started at a time when there had been difficulties in her relationship with her husband. He was a clerk in a government office. They had always got on well together, but 6 months ago he had started to be irritable and angry with her. He would not talk about why he had changed. She had not known what the problem was until a female friend had told her that he had started a relationship with a younger woman he had met at work. Odra's mother said she had been really upset and had confided in Odra's 14-year-old sister, but she could not talk to Odra about it. Now she was worried that her husband was going to leave her. He had started to spend nights away from the home, saying he had extra work to do, but she knew this was not true. She was sure that Odra's problems were caused by all the unhappiness in the home. What should the health professional do?

### 14.1.1 Information about parents' marriages and children

Most health professionals will know about the behaviour norms for marriage in their locality. In many places, however, the nature of the relationship has changed over recent years because of increasing Western influence. In all societies, no matter what the type of marriage, children have a need for continuing warmth and affection from their parents. The following are ways in which marriage varies across cultures.

### Ages of marriage

In some societies, marriage at 16 years is common; in others it is regarded as highly undesirable.

### Pre-marital relationships

In cultures where marriages are arranged, the bride and bridegroom may not have met or have met only a few times before marriage. In others, the couple may have lived together for several years and had children before they marry.

### Residence after marriage

In some cultures it is expected that the bride will go to live with her husband's family. In others it is normal for the couple to set up a home on their own.

## One or more wives

In some societies it is expected that a man will have more than one wife. In others this is totally unacceptable.

## Separate or shared roles

In some societies, married men and women live almost entirely separate lives apart from their sexual relationship. In other societies they share virtually all family tasks.

## Communication

This may be free and open or the couple may hardly communicate important factual information such as the state of their finances, let alone their feelings for each other.

## Child care

This may be shared almost equally or the mother may take responsibility for all aspects of childcare. In some societies the mother takes responsibility for boys and girls up to a certain age, after which, in the case of boys, the father takes over.

## Sources of tension

All types of marriage experience tension, nearly always centring on money, sex, the upbringing of children and other relationships. In traditional societies, the relationship between the wife and her mother-in-law is a common source of tension. In Western societies, marriage strain often arises from the isolation of the couple in cramped living conditions.

## Parental separation, divorce and death

In some societies, separation and divorce are extremely uncommon. In many Western societies, as many as 1 in 2 marriages break down before children have reached age 16 years.

Children whose parents separate have a higher rate of emotional and behaviour problems than children whose parents do not separate. If parents separate amicably and remain friendly, the risk of their children developing behaviour and emotional problems is much less than if their separation is accompanied by violent and bitter arguments. All children are affected by parental separation but the majority do not develop significant emotional and behaviour problems. It is important for children that they remain in touch with both parents unless there is a risk of abusive behaviour from one of them.

When parents separate, children often feel that they are kept in the dark and that decisions that affect them are being made without asking them what their preferences are. Children are less confused if they are kept informed but should not be burdened with having to make decisions on behalf of their parents.

Children whose parents do not separate but have frequent, violent arguments have about the same level of behaviour and emotional problems as children of parents who do separate. In thinking about whether to separate or not (and, if they do separate, what the arrangements for the children should be), parents need to ensure that their children's needs are paramount.

In societies with high adult mortality, especially those with a high prevalence of HIV infection, many children will have lost a parent through death before reaching adulthood. In others, very few children lose a parent through death before this age. Children who lose a parent by death are also affected by the loss (see Section 14.2), but the majority do not show significant behaviour and emotional problems.

## 14.1.2 Finding out about the parental marriage

When children are brought to a clinic for a behaviour, emotional or developmental problem, it is always useful to have some information about the quality of the parental marriage.

Some parents will spontaneously link their child's problem with marriage difficulties. Other parents will be more defensive and upset if it is even hinted that their marriage problems are affecting their children. To avoid upsetting and angering defensive parents, questioning along the following lines may be helpful.

'Sometimes children are upset by what is happening at home or at school. What are the sorts of things that might be upsetting your child?'

'Is there anything at home that you think might be upsetting your child?'

'All parents have their ups and downs. Does that happen to you?'

'It sounds as if you sometimes get quite angry with each other. How often does that happen?' and 'How does that affect the children when it happens?'

'It really does sound as if you get quite angry with each other. Have you ever spent some time apart?'

'Have you ever thought it would be better if you spent some time apart?'

When talking to children about their parents' marriage, one needs to be very careful not to alienate the child or the parents. If you wish to approach the subject, you might begin with one of the following.

'Sometimes things happen at home that are very difficult to talk about. I don't want you to talk about anything that might upset your mum and dad if they knew you had been talking to me about it.'

'So are there things at home that you find upsetting?'

'What sorts of things?'

'Can you talk to your mum and dad about these things?'

'How do you feel about that?'

'Would you like me to talk to your mum and dad about how you are feeling?'

Some health professionals may neither have the time nor feel they have the expertise to question along these lines. In this situation and if there is nowhere to refer such problems, a health professional could merely say something like:

'Well, it has been difficult for me to work out why your child has this problem. I am sure you know that sometimes when things are not going well at home this can be upsetting for children. You may wish to think about that when you work out what is best for your child.'

Now, given the information you have obtained, try to work out if this child's behaviour and emotional problems may be a reaction to parental marital problems. Then go on to work out a plan to help.

## 14.1.3 Helping with parental marriage problems

Health professionals may feel able to explore the quality of the parental marriage and the way this might be affecting a child who has a behaviour and emotional problem. But they are unlikely to feel able to provide expert counselling for parents whose marriages are in trouble. They should nevertheless keep in mind the following principles when talking to parents who might be thinking of separating.

- It is better for children over the age of 6 years to be kept informed of any proposed changes that might affect their lives. If possible, although they should not be inappropriately burdened with making decisions, it is always a good idea to ask their views on what should happen. This is especially the case with older children.
- Parents who are thinking of separating should be clearly told that their children will be less upset if they are able to separate in a friendly way. Their children will not do so well if the separation involves violent arguments and recriminations.
- Children whose parents separate almost always suffer from the fact that there is less money to go round. They need to have this explained to them.

Now make a list of the ways in which the health professional might be able to help Odra.

# 14.2 Grief and loss

### Case 14.2

Anga is a 9-year-old girl who is brought to the clinic by her mother because she is crying, wetting the bed and does not want to go to school. This has been going on since Anga's father was killed in an accident at work 4 months ago. He fell off scaffolding at a building site and died immediately. The other two children, an older boy and a younger girl, were both very upset initially, but they seem to have adjusted to the idea that they are not going to see their father again. Anga remains very upset. She will not talk about her feelings to her mother, who herself is finding it difficult to cope. The mother's family is trying to help, but even so, the money coming into the home is much reduced. There is enough money to eat but nothing left over for extra things such as new clothes. What should the health professional do?

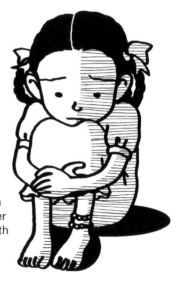

## 14.2.1 Information about grief and loss in children

Loss is a common experience in childhood. Even in high-income countries, 3 in 4 children will have experienced the death of a close relative, often a grandparent, by the age of 16. In LAMI countries with high death rates, many children will lose one or both parents by the time they reach adulthood. This is particularly likely in places where HIV/AIDS is endemic.

Loss of a parent through separation or divorce is an increasingly common experience for children in Westernised countries than the loss of a parent through death. Parental separation is also increasingly common in LAMI countries and is discussed in the previous section.

Children's ideas of death change as they get older (Clinical Center, 2006).

- Pre-school children see death as reversible and temporary – they watch cartoon characters get killed, then get up again and carry on as if nothing has happened.

- Between 5 and 9 years, children begin to realise that death is final but retain the belief that a person can come back to life. They may form an image of death in their minds, for example as an angel of death or a skeleton.
- From age 10 upwards, children increasingly understand that death is irreversible and that all living things die.

Children's ideas of death will vary greatly depending on their previous experience of death. Their ideas will also depend on the religious ideas in their society. For example, in societies that believe in reincarnation, children will have very different ideas from those living in societies in which death is regarded as final and irreversible.

Reactions to death (bereavement reactions) differ widely from society to society. Individuals within societies also differ greatly in how they react to the death of a family member. The following bereavement reactions are common features shown by children under the age of 10 years and may last from a few days to several months and include:

- Confusion over why adults are so upset, constantly questioning them
- Magical thinking – the child believes that the dead person will come back
- Sense of guilt and feeling of responsibility for the death
- Sleep disturbance, perhaps with nightmares and bed-wetting.

Over the age of 10 years, reactions may last from several days to a few months and include:

- immediate disbelief and a sense of numbness
- outbursts of weeping
- outbursts of anger, perhaps towards doctors or nurses who could not keep the dead person alive
- disturbed sleep, possibly with nightmares
- difficulties in concentrating and decline in schoolwork.

The following factors influence bereavement reactions.

- Age of the child.
- Previous experience of loss by death, for example of a pet or a friend at school.
- The reactions of others around them. If others are openly crying, children will feel better able to cry themselves. If others are holding in their emotions, children may feel they should do this too.
- Whether the death was expected, for example following chronic illness, or sudden and unexpected. People, including children, take longer to adjust to an unexpected death because they have not been able to begin to mourn before the death.
- The relationship of the child to the person who has died. Reactions will be stronger if there was a close bond between the child and the person who has died.
- The length of time since the death. Crying, sleep disturbance and inability to concentrate usually fade by 3 months and disappear by 6 months. However, this varies widely.

Children who have suffered bereavement in childhood are slightly more likely to show psychological problems, especially depression, in adulthood than those who have not been bereaved, but the differences are not great. In contrast, children whose parents have separated or divorced have a distinctly increased rate of psychological problems later on.

### 14.2.2 Finding out about bereavement reactions

- What signs of bereavement is the child showing? Note that these may involve any combination of a range of behaviours and feelings. The child may show depressive features, anxiety, irritability with outbursts of temper, anger and disobedience, aggressive behaviour, sleeping or eating problems, and decline in schoolwork.

- How long have these been present? Did they start when the person died or after a period in which the child showed little reaction?
- Was the death sudden and unexpected or did it occur after a chronic illness? Has the child been told the truth about the reasons for death? This may have been especially difficult if the person ended their own life or died of HIV/AIDS.
- What was the relationship of the child to the dead person? Was it close and positive, indifferent, or perhaps tense and hostile?
- Did the child participate in the rituals following death? Or was he excluded?
- What is the current reaction of others in the family to the bereavement? Are they still showing signs of upset? Can they talk about the dead person?
- What ideas has the child expressed about what has happened to the person after death? Are these the sorts of ideas that adults have in the society in which the child is living?
- Has the child expressed his feelings about the death? Are there people around who feel comfortable talking about the death? Is the child being shunned by friends because they do not know what to say to her?
- Are there other stresses present that the child may be reacting to? Remember that there may be factors other than the bereavement that may be affecting the child's feelings and behaviour.
- Some of this information will only emerge if it is possible to talk to the child alone. The health professional should try to talk alone to all bereaved children over the age of 8 years.

Now, given the information you have obtained, try to understand this child's grief and feeling of bereavement. Then go on to work out a plan to help.

## 14.2.3 Helping bereavement reactions in children and adolescents

This will depend very greatly on the findings made in the assessment. It is important to communicate to parents the wide range of normal bereavement reactions, and active steps to provide help will be needed if, after a few weeks, the child:

- is refusing to go to sleep
- is refusing to see her friends
- has continuing anxiety, panic attacks or phobias
- is showing a persistent decline in schoolwork
- refuses to talk about the person who has died
- is showing aggressive or very disobedient behaviour
- has taken to drinking alcohol.

The health professional should try to see the child by himself. The conversation with a child aged 8 years or over might begin:

'I know that your ......... died a few weeks ago. Could you tell me a bit about him please?'

If the child only says positive things, one might go on:

'Well, those are a lot of good things. Were there any things that were not so good? After all, no one is perfect.'

After the child has talked about the person's good and bad points, one might go on to ask: 'How did you and he get on?' and then 'What do you miss most about him?'

The conversation might then go on to deal with why the person died when they did. With parental permission, the child may need to be told the truth of what happened later on, but the health professional should not divulge such information without getting permission from the parents. How is the child currently feeling about the death? Are those feelings changing as time goes on?

It is important to find out whether the child feels responsible for the death in any way. Younger children especially may have fantasies along these lines that they find difficulty in expressing. If such fantasies exist, the child may be asked whether there is anything that might make him feel he was not to blame in some way. In addition, the parents or, if a parent has died, the surviving parent may need the opportunity to talk about their own feelings of loss.

Now make a list of the ways in which the health professional might be able to help Anga.

# 14.3 Physical abuse

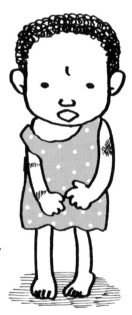

**Case 14.3**

Khalifa was brought by her mother to the health clinic in a poor part of the city one morning because, her mother said, she was not moving her left arm. The 4-year-old was crying bitterly and it was obvious that she was in pain. She screamed when her arm was touched or when the health professional tried to move it. There was a bruise on the forearm. The health professional suspected a fracture and an X-ray confirmed this. The X-ray also showed that Khalifa had old rib fractures. The mother was asked how the arm fracture had occurred and said she did not really know. She also did not know how the rib fractures had come about. Khalifa must have fallen. The mother looked uncomfortable when she gave her explanation. The bruise stretched right round the arm and it looked as if someone had gripped the arm very tightly. Neither the fracture nor the bruise looked as if they could have been caused by a fall. The health professional noticed that Khalifa was very thin and looked dirty and uncared for. She had no difficulty in deciding that Khalifa was both neglected and the victim of physical abuse. What should the health professional do?

## 14.3.1 Information about physical abuse

Physical abuse occurs when an adult inflicts a physical injury on a child to a degree that is unacceptable in the society in which the family lives.

What is regarded as acceptable physical punishment varies between societies. In some societies it is acceptable for parents and teachers to beat children extremely hard when they see them as being naughty or disobedient. Indeed in some places it is thought that to be a good parent it is necessary to beat your child for bad behaviour. On the other hand, some places it is against the law for parents (or teachers) to hit children when they are naughty.

Physical abuse occurs across the social spectrum, even in very rich families, where it may be inflicted by parents or servants. However, it is far more common in poor families, living on the edge, where parents are experiencing multiple stresses. Such practices can cause both physical and psychological harm to the child.

Even in societies where physical punishment, even severe physical punishment, is 'normal', children who are beaten are more likely to be aggressive and anxious later on in life than those who are disciplined in other ways.

Unless the injury is very minor (scratches or small, single bruises), health professionals should regard the presence of all physical injury for which the parents cannot provide a convincing explanation as evidence of physical abuse. The following injuries are likely to be signs of physical abuse:

- bruising on the face, ear lobes, buttocks or back, especially if multiple
- crescent shape discolouration in the shape of a human bite
- burns, cigarette butt marks or scalds
- retinal haemorrhages, usually caused by head-shaking
- bone fractures for which no convincing explanation can be provided
- torn upper lip.

Conversely, bruises over the shins of toddlers and young children are common 'play bruises' and usually not associated with maltreatment. Accidental bruises are found most over bony prominences and the front of the body.

Parents who abuse their children tend to be:

- young
- unemployed
- violent and impulsive
- drinking alcohol excessively or using drugs
- the result of a violent upbringing themselves.

Characteristics of children who are abused include:

- hyperactivity
- oppositional
- have a difficult temperament
- frightened
- distrustful of adults.

Parental attitudes to the child may reveal an abusive relationship. The parents may:

- blame or belittle the child
- treat the child as a scapegoat, for example holding him responsible for all that goes wrong in the family
- be unconcerned about the child's welfare
- fail to keep appointments made for the child.

The young child may react in several ways. He may:

- become sad and withdrawn
- be suspicious of all adults
- cry and refuse food
- lose weight or fail to gain weight.

Older children may:

- become miserable and depressed
- become aggressive and violent
- fail in schoolwork
- run away from home, perhaps to the city or to other relatives.

## 14.3.2 Finding out more about a child who may have been physically abused

Information may be forthcoming from teachers, neighbours or health professionals who may notice injuries to the child, or from the child himself who may report to teachers or others that he is being physically abused.

Absolute certainty is never possible but health professionals, in making this judgement, need to be convinced that it is highly probable that the child has been physically abused.

There are a few physical conditions which, on rare occasions, may provide explanations of physical injuries that look as if they are the result of abuse but are in fact caused by something else.

- Multiple bruising may be caused by blood clotting disorders. In this case the child will probably have experienced abnormal bleeding in other circumstances such as with accidental cuts or a tooth extraction.
- Multiple fractures may be caused by very rare bone disorders, especially brittle bone disease or osteogenesis imperfecta. In this case the child will almost certainly have been brought to the clinic previously by the parents because of fractures caused by very minor injury.

A child whose injuries suggest that he has been physically abused should be examined unclothed from head to toe for signs of physical injury other than those with which the child has presented. If facilities exist, an X-ray of the whole body should also be taken. All this information should be carefully recorded, with drawings of all injuries that are visible.

The health professional who learns that a child has probably been abused, should pass this information on to the local child protection agency, usually a social worker or the police.

If there is no such agency available, then the health professional will need to take the responsibility herself. She will begin by interviewing the child. It will sometimes be a difficult task to decide whether to inform the parents before interviewing the child, because if it is the case that the abuse has taken place in the home, the parents may threaten the child and prevent him from telling the truth. In these circumstances, the health professional may be at risk of injury from family members who are angry at what they believe is an accusation against them. Health professionals therefore need to be cautious in what they say and make sure, if at all possible, that they do not act without discussion with whoever is in charge of the clinic.

If, as happens occasionally, it seems likely that abuse has occurred outside the family or that no family member has been involved, then the health professional should tell the parents that she needs to talk to the child with a parent present as the possibility exists that the child has been abused. If a family member has been involved, then tell the parents that you need to talk to the child. Someone known to the child but who is not family, such as a teacher, should be present.

Many children who have been physically abused will, in fact, be too young to interview. Children over the age of 4 years should, however, be interviewed. When interviewing children at risk of abuse with or without a parent present:

- make sure that you put the child at ease before asking difficult questions – you can use toys or drawing or talk about neutral subjects such as things the child enjoys doing or subjects the child enjoys at school;
- speak calmly and ask questions without putting any ideas into the child's head;
- do not accuse anyone in the child's presence;

- ask questions such as 'Sometimes children can get hurt by a grown-up. Has that happened to you?' If the child answers positively, go on to ask 'Please could you let me know who has been hurting you?', then go on to ask what happened and if the child has told anyone else about this;
- when the extent of the child's injuries is known, the parent(s) may be asked questions such as: 'X has got these [describe injuries]. How do you think this happened?';
- assuming an inadequate or unconvincing explanation is given: 'It doesn't seem to me that that could explain the injury. Have you any other ideas how it could have occurred?' or 'Is there anyone else in the home who would be able to tell me more?' or 'I'm afraid it looks to me as if X has been hit by someone. Have you any idea who that could be?'

The health professional may then go on to try to give the parent or the person who has brought the child the opportunity to express their feelings. You can say things such as: 'This must be very upsetting for you. How do you feel about the fact that X is hurt and you don't seem to be able to explain this?' Given this opportunity, the adult responsible is more likely to be open and honest about what has really occurred.

Always make sure that you write down exactly what both parents and children have said as soon as they have talked to you.

## 14.3.3 Helping children who have been physically abused

Once it is clear that a child has been physically abused, what the health professional should do depends on whether there is a child protection service in the area. If such a service exists, then the health professional should immediately alert the service to the problem. In most places the presence of a child protection service will also mean that the police will have to be involved. In these circumstances the role of the health professional is to make sure that the problem is being dealt with by the child protection service and that this service has all the information it needs to make the best decisions on behalf of the child. If a child protection service is available, the health professional has two tasks:

1   to establish that the child's injuries have been caused by unexplained trauma
2   to keep the child safe until the child protection service can take over.

If a child protection service does not exist, then the health professional will need to take responsibility for ensuring that the child is as well protected and receives the best possible care.

## 14.3.4 Principles of good care for a child who has been abused

- The child needs to be safe from further abuse. This is the number one priority but remember it is never possible to guarantee absolute safety.
- The child should remain in as familiar a place as possible, preferably the home, as long as it is safe to do so. In Western countries, children who had been abused were, until quite recently, removed from their homes. It is now realised that the removal from loved ones is often more harmful than keeping children at home.
- All family members should be involved in taking responsibility for the child's welfare. Grandparents may have a particularly important part to play, especially as the parents are likely to be young.
- The family should be treated with respect; horror at what has occurred should not result in rudeness to or rejection of family members.
- If the family is prepared to accept help from them, local resources such as voluntary organisations that help families should be involved.

- The fact that the child has been abused and requires to be kept safe should not draw attention away from all the other needs the child is likely to have, such as for adequate nutrition, healthcare, clothes, stimulation and education.

### 14.3.5 Helping the abused child

Helping the abused child can take a number of forms (Box 14.1). However, remember it is not just the child who will need help. Other family members may also be under stress. They should be given the opportunity to talk and help should be provided depending on their needs. If a family member has been involved, it may be necessary for this member to leave the family at least for a period of time.

Once the abuse has been made known, the person responsible may stop it, but this does not always happen. The child should be given the opportunity over the following weeks and months to say whether he is still being hurt, physically, sexually or otherwise.

Continuing abuse may mean that the child will need to be found an alternative home. If at all possible this should be with a relative (e.g. aunt, grandparent), but where no family member is prepared to take on the responsibility, then the child may need to be placed in a children's home or orphanage. If at all possible, contact with the family should be maintained.

Now write down the ways in which you think a health professional could help Khalifa.

---

Box 14.1 Helping the abused child

1 Help the child feel positive about himself
   - Reassure the child that he is not responsible for the abuse
   - Give positive messages to the child about his behaviour and emotions
   - Suggest activities that the child enjoys, such as playing with friends
2 Help the child to trust
   - Be someone who the child can talk to in confidence
   - Spend time alone with the child
   - Show love and affection, but remember to be careful about physical touching
3 Help the child to identify and express emotions
   - Play games that involve feelings and emotions
   - Read books that involve emotions
   - Talk about what emotions the child is experiencing and why
   - Teach the child ways of dealing with anger, such as playing with toys until he calms down
4 Help the child make a safety plan
   - If there is a local police number, write it down somewhere where the child will find it easily
   - Choose a friend or neighbour where the child can go for help
   - Help the child to say 'no' to the adult
5 Healing messages for children
   - I care about you
   - I respect you
   - You are lovable
   - You have strengths
   - It is a good thing you have told me; now we can try hard to make sure you will not be hurt again
   - Most adults would never hurt children
   - You can say 'no' if you do not like the way someone touches you.

Patel (2003)

---

## 14.4 Sexual abuse

**Case 14.4**

Soraya is a 5-year-old girl who is brought to the clinic by her mother with a stomach ache in the lower part of her abdomen. On examining her, the health professional notices that there is bruising around the vulva. When she gently parts the vulva she notices also that there is a tear inside the vulva and that the girl has a vaginal discharge. What should the health professional do?

### 14.4.1 Information about sexual abuse

Sexual abuse has occurred when children and young adolescents are involved in sexual activities with adults or older adolescents with or without their consent. Such activities may involve sexual contact such as penetration of the vagina or anus, or lesser forms of sexual activity such as fondling of the genitalia. Another form of sexual abuse involves the making of films or videos of children participating in sexual activities. Non-contact abuse occurs when, for example, a man 'exhibits' his penis to a child while masturbating. Penetrative abuse is often preceded by a period of 'grooming' when the older man begins by befriending and then stroking and fondling other parts of the child's body before moving on to the genitalia. Both boys and girls can be victims of sexual abuse.

Sexual abuse has certainly or almost certainly occurred when:

- a child under the age of consent (14 or 16 years in most countries) has physical signs of sexual contact – perforated hymen, bruising or cuts in or around the vulva, damage to the anus or a sexually transmitted infection such as chlamydia or gonorrhoea. It is important to remember though that many forms of sexual abuse can occur without any abnormalities being found on physical examination;
- a child of this age reports that he is being sexually molested. It is very unusual for children of this age to make up such stories and they should be assumed to be telling the truth unless there is very good evidence to the contrary.

Sexual abuse should be suspected if there is:

- precocious sexualised behaviour, but remember that this type of behaviour may be shown by many other children who are influenced by media portrayal of sexually aware children
- touching and playing with sexual parts in public.

Sexual abuse should be borne in mind as a possibility when a child shows any of a range of behaviour and emotional problems for which there is no convincing explanation. The health professional should, however, be very reluctant to assume abuse has occurred without the presence of more positive evidence.

If the perpetrator is a child or adolescent, it is important to remember that they too may be a victim. Overwhelmingly, sexual abuse is perpetrated by older boys and men on younger boys and girls. However, women are also sometimes perpetrators. The perpetrator has often been abused himself as a child and in adulthood he often has problems with excessive alcohol consumption or is using illegal drugs.

Most sexual abuse is carried out by family members. Fathers or stepfathers are often involved. If the father is the perpetrator, the mother may sometimes know about what is going on but may say nothing because of fear. In addition, there are often other forms of family violence occurring at the same time. For example, the mother may herself be the victim of domestic violence. Sexual abuse by strangers outside the family is much less common, although when it occurs it is much more widely publicised.

Children who are victims of sexual abuse may become sad and withdrawn, show aggressive behaviour problems, fail in their schoolwork or run away from home. These problems may, however, arise from any severe stress and it should not be assumed that the child has been the victim of abuse without strong confirming evidence.

## 14.4.2 Finding out more about a child when sexual abuse is suspected

When sexual abuse is suspected, the assessment will depend on the availability of specialist resources. In some areas there will be a Social Services department to carry out the assessment. In many places there will not even be a social worker to advise. The health professional will then have to depend on his own skills and on the limited local resources that are available.

First, it should be explained to the parents that there is reason to think that their child has been sexually 'interfered with'. If the parents have brought the possibility of sexual abuse to attention, this will, of course, not be necessary.

After an explanation to the child at a level appropriate to the child's understanding, there should be a general physical examination with the mother present (if this is not appropriate, then with another familiar person), followed by examination of the external genitalia for signs of injury. If there is a discharge and if facilities exist, a specimen should be taken for culture. All observations should be carefully recorded, with drawings of any injuries noted. Examination of the genitals for signs of sexual abuse can be difficult, especially if the damage is relatively slight. If possible this should be done by someone who is experienced in this type of work.

In most places there will be no child protection team available to deal with child abuse cases. In these cases the health professional needs to begin by interviewing the parent(s). She will begin by explaining that there is a concern that someone has been hurting the child's 'private parts'. She will explain that this is a very serious matter and that she will have to ask some difficult questions. She can then find out from the parent what the family names for the genitalia are. She may ask:

'What do you call the part of X's body where she does her wee?' and 'What does X call that part of her body?'

This will give the health professional a shared vocabulary with family members, including the child. She may then go on to ask the mother:

'It looks as if there has been some interference with X's private parts [or whatever word the mother has used]. I wonder how you think this could have happened?' and 'Who do you think could have done this?'

If the mother reveals she has been aware of what has been going on, she will need to be asked what she has done about it and who else she has told. The mother's response should be carefully recorded.

If at all possible and if the child is over the age of 4 years, the health professional should ask permission from the mother to talk to the child separately, explaining that some children find it easier to talk when they are alone. The child should be put at ease before moving on to ask for details of the abuse. At this point the health professional can begin by asking the child to make a drawing of the body. Alternatively, the health professional can draw a body and then point to the genital area and ask:

'What do you call that part of you, down there?'

'Has anyone touched your [term the child has used]?'

'Did you like that, or not very much?'

'Did it hurt?'

'Who did that?'

'Did you ask them to stop?'

(In specialist facilities there will probably be a number of anatomically correct dolls to make communication easier, but these are unlikely to be available to most health professionals).

The child's answers may make clear what has been going on and who has been responsible. On the other hand, many children who have been sexually abused will deny this has happened because they know it is wrong and do not want to get the perpetrator into trouble. Whatever the child has said the health professional will need to record.

Now, given the information you have obtained, try to understand why this child is being sexually abused. Then go on to work out a plan to help.

## 14.4.3 How to help children who have probably or definitely been sexually abused

Once it is clear that a child has probably or definitely been sexually abused, what the health professional should do depends on whether there is a child protection service in the area. If such a service exists, then the health professional should immediately alert the service to the problem. In most places the presence of a child protection service will also mean that the police will have to be involved. In these circumstances the role of the health professional is to make sure that the problem is being dealt with by the child protection service and that this service has all the information it needs to make the best decisions on behalf of the child.

If a child protection service is available, the health professional has two tasks:

1    to establish that the child has been probably or definitely sexually abused
2    to keep the child safe until the child protection service can take over.

If a child protection service does not exist, then the health professional will need to take responsibility for ensuring that the child is well protected and receives as good care as is possible.

The same principles apply to the care of children who have been sexually abused as with those who have been physically abused (see Section 14.3).

Health professionals who identify sexual abuse may be at risk of injury from family members who are angry at what they think is an accusation against them. Health professionals therefore need to be cautious in what they say and make sure, if at all possible, that they do not act without discussion with whoever is in charge of the clinic.

Now write down ways in which a health professional could help Soraya.

## 14.5 Emotional abuse

**Case 14.5**

Nikhil is a 7-year-old boy brought to the clinic because he is wetting the bed. In fact he only wets the bed about once a month and the health professional does not think this needs any special treatment. But she notices that while the mother is talking about Nikhil she seems to be extremely angry with him. She says the bed-wetting is just one of the ways in which Nikhil tries to hurt her. He never does anything to help in the home. Compared with his 10-year-old sister, he is 'useless'. When Nikhil tries to speak she shuts him up immediately. The health professional asks what are the good things about Nikhil, and the mother says 'Well, there isn't much good about him. Oh yes, he does once in a while give some sweets to his sister, but he only does that because he wants something from her.' The health professional feels this mother really dislikes her son. What should the health professional do?

### 14.5.1 Information about emotional abuse

In this type of abuse the child is damaged not by physical injury but by a combination of rejection and lack of affection. Emotional abuse is nearly always accompanied by neglect (see Section 14.6). It may be shown in a number of ways. The child may be:

- exposed to relentless criticism and hostility from one or both parents
- deprived of affection – there will be no warmth shown to the child in the way of praise or cuddles or hugs
- ignored – when the child tries to draw attention to something he has done, he is ignored or told off
- exposed to threats – the child is, for example, frequently told he will be sent away from home
- exposed to stressful situations he is in no position to influence – for example, the child may witness his father beating up his mother without anyone caring to think about what he must feel.

Emotional abuse is often linked to:

- poor social circumstances (although many children living in poverty are in no way emotionally abused; on the other hand, some children living in affluent homes may be emotionally abused by servants, relatives living in the home or parents who are absorbed with their own lives and have little time for their children)
- living in a disadvantaged neighbourhood, with high rates of violence and unemployment
- parental problems, when parents:
  - have often had a harsh upbringing themselves
  - are violent and impulsive
  - show excessive alcohol consumption
  - use illegal drugs
  - punish harshly
- behaviour problems – the child may:
  - have a difficult temperament
  - be excessively demanding
  - be frequently disobedient.

A child may be singled out or made a scapegoat, while other siblings are appropriately loved and emotionally supported. This may be due to parental attitudes relating to the past. For example, the child may be:

- not of the gender the parent wanted
- conceived by a partner from a different relationship – often a secret held by the mother
- born at the wrong time, disrupting parental plans
- have an intellectual disability or a physical disability
- have a personality that conflicts with that of one parent.

## 14.5.2 Finding out more about a child who is being emotionally abused

The health professional should look out for:

- the possibility that the child has undiagnosed developmental problems (intellectual disability, a specific delay, hyperactivity, ASD) that may make parenting more difficult (note that some of these problems may have arisen as a result of emotional abuse and not be the cause of it);
- constant belittling of the child, who cannot do anything right; if the child does something positive the parent may say, for example, that she cannot remember the last time he did this;
- a lack of warmth in the parent's tone of voice when talking to or about the child;
- parents giving the impression that the child is always trying to irritate or annoy them.

All these behaviours are likely to be even more damaging if the child is singled out for hostile or rejecting behaviour, while other children receive more favourable treatment.

Now, given the information you have obtained, try to understand why this child is being emotionally abused. Then go on to work out a plan to help.

## 14.5.3 How to help a child who is being emotionally abused

Action to reduce emotional abuse could involve:

- talking to the parents about the child's need for love and affection
- showing caring behaviour to the parents and trying to find out at least the small, positive ways they are behaving towards their child
- if the child does have a developmental problem, discussing this with the parents in such a way to help them to both promote development and rebuild affection towards the child
- a discussion with teachers or other relatives
- working out ways of helping the child to spend time away from the family, with neighbours, friends or other relatives
- giving the child the opportunity to talk about his feelings at being rejected and sympathising with him, making it clear he is not alone in the world.

Now write down ways the health professional could help Nikhil.

# 14.6 Neglect

**Case 14.6**

Maya is an 18-month-old girl in an orphanage. She has been in the orphanage since the age of 3 months when her mother became unable to look after her because she had AIDS. Her mother died 2 months later. Her father died of AIDS while her mother was pregnant with her. There were no grandparents or other relatives available to take over her care. No one from the family came to visit Maya. A health professional who visited the orphanage on a regular basis was asked to see Maya because the staff were worried about her and wondered whether she had a physical illness. She

163

found Maya lying in a cot with the sides up in the middle of the afternoon. The staff of the orphanage said they were so short of staff that no one was available to take her out into the garden. They told the health professional that there was no one who took a particular interest in Maya. One member of staff had spent a lot of time with Maya after she was admitted to the orphanage but this person had left about a month ago. Shortly afterwards Maya had started to refuse most foods. She seemed lacking in energy and was listless. When the health professional spoke to her she did not respond, but just lay in her cot. There did not seem to be anything physically the matter with her. What should the health professional do?

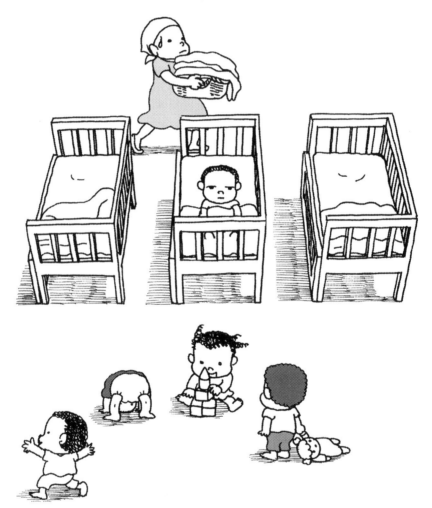

**Case 14.7**

Maliki is a 6-year-old girl who has been sent to a health clinic by the school because her teachers think she is very small for her age and they are worried about her. She comes with her mother. When she is weighed and measured, Maliki is below the third centile for height. Her mother is also small and very quiet. It is difficult to hear her speak. It turns out she has six children and Maliki is the youngest. Her mother has no complaints about Maliki. She says she is such a good girl that she often forgets she is there. The girl looks unwashed and is wearing clothes with holes in them. The health professional has seen other children in this family and knows they are better looked after.

## 14.6.1 Information about children who are neglected

In this form of maltreatment no actions are taken that harm the child. Instead, the child is denied essential care that all children should receive. This can be just as, if not more, harmful than more active forms of abuse. There are several types of neglect, which may occur together.

- Lack of physical care. The child is likely to appear dirty, undernourished and has inadequate clothing. Poor parents will not be able to provide their children with new, smart clothes, but most will manage to ensure that their children are dressed in clean clothes, even if they are shabby.
- Lack of warm, affectionate care. Children do not receive hugs and cuddles and are rarely, if ever, praised when they have performed well.
- Lack of supervision to ensure safety. Children are allowed to play in dangerous areas, for example around busy roads where they are at risk of being victims of road traffic accidents. Parents often do not know where their children are playing and there are no rules about the time they are expected to come in from playing outside in the evening or when they are expected to be in bed.
- Lack of stimulation to promote learning and development of intelligence. The parents show no interest in helping their children to learn. They do not make sure they attend school regularly. They do not read to their children or listen to them reading.
- Lack of healthcare. Parents neglect the presence of major or minor illness, not taking their children to health professionals when clearly they are in need of medical or nursing attention.

Causes of neglect include:

- lack of money
- unemployment
- large numbers of children
- poor household organisation
- young parents
- parents with mild intellectual disability
- parents who have been neglected in their own childhood
- parental, especially maternal, depression or other mental disorders
- issues relating to emotional abuse (see Section 14.5).

The impact it has on the child includes:

- failure to thrive, physically or emotionally
- small stature
- mild intellectual disability
- failure in schoolwork
- lack of close attachment to parents
- overfriendly relationships with strangers.

## 14.6.2 Finding out more about a child who may be neglected

The identification of child neglect does not usually present many problems provided the possibility that it is present is borne in mind. Observation of the mother and child will usually prove quite sufficient to establish whether a child is being neglected.

The child should be physically examined and all the findings, especially the height and weight of the child, should be recorded.

Some assessment of the child's level of mental function should also be made in terms of the child's mental age. Are the child's replies to questions like that of a child of his actual age or are the replies more like that of a child 1, 2 or even 3 years younger?

Now, given the information you have obtained, try to understand why this child is being neglected. Then go on to work out a plan to help.

### 14.6.3 How to help a child who is neglected

The parents should be given as much help as possible to improve their care of the child. If the parents are experiencing stress themselves, providing help may give them more ability to care for their child. Relatives, neighbours, friends or local community support might be recruited to support the parents, perhaps take over some of the childcare and thus improve the child's quality of life. Advice to parents and relatives might include:

- advice on the child's diet
- help to obtain more food for the child
- advice on how to show physical affection to the child
- advice on how to keep the child safe
- encouragement to send the child to school regularly, monitoring the child's school attendance
- explanation of how to bring the child to a clinic for check-ups and for medical or nursing care if the child is ill.

If health professionals are involved with children in orphanages who are neglected, they should use their influence to improve the conditions in the institution. This might involve encouragement to ensure:

- a better staff to child ratio, with more adults looking after each child
- more personalised care, with children being allocated special caregivers who will be responsible for their care
- stimulation appropriate for the developmental level of the child
- good healthcare and nutrition
- an active programme to transfer the children to good family care, with either an adoption or long-term fostering arrangement.

Now describe how a health professional might be able to help Maya and Maliki.

## 14.7 Children in disasters

**Case 14.8**

A health professional is contacted and asked to go to a large village in a rural area 50 miles away from where she works. The village, with a population of a 1000 people of whom 300 were children, was devastated by a landslide a week ago. In the car on the way she is told that most of the houses in the village were destroyed and the rest have been deemed unsafe. About 100 people were killed and a number of others injured. The surviving members of the village have been housed in tents in a camp that has been set up 5 miles from the landslide area. The camp is being supplied with clean water and a sufficient supply of food. The injured, another 100 people, have been taken to a hospital in a city 100 miles away. The health professional is told that she is to take responsibility for the welfare of the children in the camp. What should be going through her mind about what she is going to do as she nears the village?

## 14.7.1 Information about the needs of children who are victims of disasters

When disasters occur, individuals experience feelings of helplessness and hopelessness. Feelings of confusion about what has happened are mixed with feelings of loss. The sooner the community regains a sense of empowerment over its own future, the more rapidly will its members come to terms with what has happened, so it is important that decision-making becomes the responsibility of the community leaders and the rest of the population as soon as possible.

The paramount need of children who have become victims of disaster is to be reunited with their parents if they are still alive and with substitute parents who will take responsibility for them if the parents have died. Similarly, the paramount need of parents is to be reunited with their children. In most disasters involving loss of life and serious injury, separation of children from parents occurs because the injured child/parent is removed from the scene for emergency, life-saving treatment.

The most common mental health consequence of both natural and man-made disasters is PTSD (see Section 14.8). However, reactions to sudden overwhelming stress may include the whole range of emotional and behaviour disorders.

## 14.7.2 Assessment of children's needs in a disaster area

The first requirement is to identify and obtain names for all the children under 16 years in the affected area and in hospital or emergency treatment centres. This should be done by the leading aid organisation together with the community leaders. The second requirement is to identify those children who are separated from their parents. Attempts should also be made to keep all family members, especially brothers and sisters, together. Questions that should be asked are:

- Are the physical needs (e.g. food and water, clothing and shelter) of the children being met?
- Have all physical injuries been attended to?
- Have all children had the opportunity, if they wish to take it, of describing what happened to them and what their main worries and anxieties are at the present time?
- What practical steps are necessary to re-establish normal life, including attendance at school classes?

Now, using the information you have obtained about the disaster and the way the child and family have been involved, try to understand how they are feeling. Then decide what is the best course of action.

## 14.7.3 Treatment of children who have been exposed to disaster

Assuming that all the physical needs of the child population have been met, and that family members have been reunited as best as possible, the next step is to ensure that the mental health needs of the children are considered.

Engaging children in activities aimed at restoring normal life will give them a sense of responsibility and self-esteem. Children should be involved in tasks such as helping adults to obtain and carry food and water, putting up tents, looking after younger children, etc., as much as possible. In addition, give all children with PTSD or other emotional reactions appropriate intervention (see Section 14.8), using activities such as drawing, colouring and group work.

Now make a list of the ways in which health professionals called to disaster areas can most helpfully meet the mental health needs of children.

## 14.8 Post-traumatic stress

**Case 14.9**

Shakiri is a 7-year-old girl brought by her mother to the clinic. About a year ago, a heater in their home caught fire and the shack in which the family lived was burned down. Shakiri, her parents and her 9-year-old brother were able to get out but her baby sister, aged 9 months, who was sleeping near the heater, was badly burned and died shortly afterwards. The family went to live with a relative but have now found another shack to live in. Although Shakiri's parents and brother were very upset for some months, they are now able to get on with their lives, but since that time Shakiri tells her mother that she cannot stop thinking about the fire and about her baby sister. She wakes several times during the night, crying out for her mother. Previously, she could happily play outside with other children, but now she cannot bear to let her mother out of her sight. When she plays at home, her mother can see she is constantly going over the events of the fire. She will not go anywhere near to where the shack was burned down. She is too frightened to go to school. What can the health professional do?

### 14.8.1 Information about post-traumatic stress

Post-traumatic stress (stress following trauma) can occur after any natural or man-made disaster affecting large groups of people. Natural disasters include earthquakes, volcanic eruptions, floods, tsunamis and bush fires. Man-made disasters include wars, civil disturbances and train crashes. Children may also experience post-traumatic stress reactions following sexual or physical abuse, or sudden, unexpected separation from their parents.

Stress reactions following trauma can take the following forms.

- Flashbacks or sudden acutely frightening feelings that the traumatic event is happening again and that one is reliving it – this is unusual in young children but more common in adolescents
- Sleep disturbances such as difficulty in getting to sleep, waking during the night, nightmares and sleep-walking
- Difficulties in separating from parents
- Difficulties in concentration and memory
- Avoidance of the place where the trauma occurred
- In teenagers, aggressive and risk-taking behaviour.

These reactions are very common after an acutely traumatic event, occurring in as many as a third of disaster victims. These reactions usually reduce in intensity over time. In about a third of those who experience such symptoms, they disappear by the end of a year. In some children, however, they persist well beyond this time.

Children who are not separated from their parents and are well supported by them after the trauma, have friends to talk to, and do not regard themselves as in any way responsible for the traumatic event are much less likely to develop a stress reaction of this sort. Children who have suffered trauma at the hands of a family member are more likely to have persistent, disabling symptoms.

### 14.8.2 Finding out more about children with post-traumatic stress

- Find out the details of the trauma to which the child has been exposed. In what way was the child involved?
- What symptoms is the child is showing? How severe are they and in what way are they interfering with the child's life?

- How soon after the trauma did the child first show these symptoms?
- Has the child had an opportunity to talk about the trauma and how he was involved?
- Has the child been separated from parents and other familiar figures?
- What was the child's personality before exposure to the trauma?
- Are there stresses other than the traumatic event to which the child has been exposed? For example, has he been exposed to quarrelling between his parents or bullying at school?
- How have the parents responded to the symptoms the child is showing?
- How does the child think of the traumatic event? Does he think of himself as responsible in any way? Who does the child think is responsible?
- Identify any mistaken beliefs the child may have about the likely recurrence of the trauma.
- Identify any stimuli that may bring back the fears of the child, for example the presence of a well-controlled bonfire making the child think his house is going to get burned down again or a low-flying aeroplane making the child think there is going to be another plane crash.
- Do any other members of the family have post-traumatic stress symptoms? How are these being handled?
- Has the child been involved in any way in restoring any damage caused by the traumatic event?
- Is the stress reaction getting worse or better?

Now, using the information you have obtained about the post-traumatic stress and the reactions of the child and family since that time, try to understand why the child has problems at this time. Then decide what is the best course of action.

## 14.8.3 Helping children with post-traumatic stress

- Give the child and parents an opportunity to talk about the traumatic experience, separately and together. Do not try to force children to talk about their experiences if they do not want to. The child can be given drawing or painting materials. Given this opportunity, the child may choose to draw or paint the stressful event.
- Explain to the parents and to the child (if of a suitable age) that it is very common for children who have been exposed to trauma to have these types of symptoms. This aims to make the child and parents less ashamed.
- Discuss any mistaken beliefs the child may have about the likely recurrence of the traumatic experience.
- Help the child to think of stimuli that seem to bring back the traumatic event in a more normal way. For example, help the child to think of the sound of a low-flying plane in a different way than in terms of another crash. You might, for example, get the child to keep a record of when he hears a plane and what happens afterwards.
- With young children suggest they play out the traumatic event with a non-traumatic conclusion. For example, the child may be helped to play out a scene in which there is a flood and people are able to get away.
- Involve parents in all procedures of this type.
- If there are several children experiencing post-traumatic stress, you can see them all together in a group to apply these techniques.
- Do not use medication for this type of problem as there is a lack of evidence for its effectiveness and the child may become habituated to such medication or experience unpleasant side-effects.

- Try to make sure children and adolescents are involved in actions to repair damage after an event or to prevent a recurrence.

Now make a list of the ways in which the health professional might be able to help Shakiri.

# CHAPTER 15

# Parents and the needs of children

Health professionals are sometimes asked to give talks to groups of parents, especially mothers, in the community in which they work. They may be requested, for example, to give a talk on the needs of children and how they can best be met.

Parents who come to these talks will often have their own very definite ideas about the upbringing of children, so health professionals may find that it makes for a good introduction to ask mothers first to describe, for example, what are the most important things for parents to do when bringing up their children, what are the mistakes most often made and how best these can be avoided. There are great differences between societies in the way children are brought up. If a health professional encourages parents to express their own views first, she will be in a better position later on in the session to relate her own views to those of her audience. All the same, children's needs are similar throughout the world. What follows is information about these needs.

## 15.1 Basic physical care

Children first need enough nutritious food and drink to enable them to grow. They need to be kept warm in cold climates and protected from the sun in hot climates.

## 15.2 Secure sense of attachment

Attachment is a bond of affection between the infant and the main caregiver(s). The bond is reciprocal between the child and the caregiver. It has arisen to meet the child's need for safety, security and protection. It is a process in which both caregiver (usually the mother) and babies play an active part. Attachment, occurring similarly in all societies in both high-income and LAMI countries, unfolds in the following way.

- Although it is not easy to observe, babies can in fact tell the difference between their own mother and other people from the first few days of life.
- At the same time, the main caregiver develops a strong sense of affection or love for the baby.
- By 6 months of age, the infant is smiling in response to familiar faces. At this point the baby develops a more active and easily observed interest in special people. It is at this stage of development that the baby is distressed if separated from its main caregiver. The intensity of attachment tends to be strongest towards people who spend time with the child and give affection – usually the mother and other members of the family. Fears also begin to develop now, first to unexpected sounds or sights and later to specific situations such as darkness.

- At about 8 months, babies show fear of strangers and may panic if someone approaches them too quickly (stranger anxiety). This usually disappears in a few months.
- Between the ages of 1 and 2 years, a specific pattern of attachment develops with the people who are looking after the child, i.e. the primary attachment figure(s). In some societies the child's attachment is strongly focused on the mother; in others where childcare is more widely shared, attachment develops between a number of caregivers and the child. The pattern will depend on the early experiences of the child. Various patterns have been described.
  - A warm, supportive and interactive relationship between the infant and the mother (or the mother and the other people who are mainly responsible for bringing up the child) leads to the development of a secure attachment. The child is distressed when separated from its caregiver, but because he learns to trust that the caregiver will return, he is gradually able to tolerate longer and longer periods of separation. This is a universal finding.
  - Overprotective parents, frequent separations, frequent change of home environment and carers, an unusually sensitive temperament in the baby and an insecure environment can combine to form a poor or insecure attachment. This may result in later emotional difficulties as well as feeding problems and failure to thrive (see Section 6.1). Lack of stimulation and failure to provide adequate care and nutrition (see Section 14.6 on neglect) can also lead to developmental problems.

## 15.3 Love and affection

This is a most important ingredient in the upbringing of children. It seems so simple – of course children need love. But there are complications. Should love be unconditional? Should parents love their children no matter what they do? Yes, to a degree. A parent can and indeed should disapprove of behaviour that is wrong and perhaps punish the child if necessary, but this should not stop parents continuing to love their children. But love does not necessarily come just because it is ordered, so one needs to know the conditions that result in parents being able to provide their children with enduring love. What are these conditions?

- Parents who love each other, support each other emotionally and do not repeatedly argue with each other are more likely to be able to love their children unconditionally.
- Parents who are not stressed by financial hardship, fears of unemployment or other stresses are more likely to be able to give their children the love they need.
- Parents who are physically and mentally well are more likely to be able to love their children.

From love comes the mutual attachment described above, with the child being unhappy when separated from the parent and the parent having the same feeling about the child. Gradually, the child feels safe even when the parent is not present. Much learning about feelings occurs within this attachment relationship.

### Safety and security

Elsewhere in this manual we describe the way many children experience physical, sexual and emotional abuse as well as neglect. Most such abuse arises within the home, inflicted by parents or other family members, so a child's safety and security largely depend on what happens in this environment. Safety from uncontrolled anger of parents, safety from sexual feelings that other family members may have for young children, and safety from the humiliation to which some parents expose their children by teasing or belittling are indicators of how children need to be kept safe. Of course there are also risks outside the home, including physical risks from road traffic, agricultural machinery, poisons and medicines that should be kept well away from young children.

## 15.4 Age-appropriate stimulation

A child's learning begins in the very first few weeks of life and communication between mothers and children begins well before the first signs of the understanding of spoken language appear. Play is the way young children learn. If they have the opportunity to play with their parents as well as their friends, this will improve their capacity to learn. The following are useful ways in which parents can provide stimulation for their children.

- Talk to your child about what you are doing.
- Ask him to tell you what he is doing.
- Ask him what, for example, a cup or a spoon is used for.
- Help him to learn what words like 'up' and 'down', 'over' and 'under', 'above' and 'below' mean.
- Help him to make comparisons, such as 'Where is the biggest tree?'
- Playing games with children and talking at the same time is a good way to encourage language development. Going shopping provides many opportunities for this too.
- Try to make watching television an active experience by making sure the child talks about what he sees.
- Telling stories to the child is more likely to help language development if he is engaged in adding to the story or (if it is a familiar story) recounting what is going to happen next.
- Reading to children and, later, listening to children reading and then talking to them about what has been read is an excellent way to improve their vocabulary.
- Watching television may be a rather passive form of entertainment, but if parents talk to children about programmes they have both watched, this again stimulates learning.

We have listed many other tips in Section 4.2.3 when discussing the needs of children with language delay. However, all children need this type of stimulation.

## 15.5 Guidance and control

One of the basic traditional roles of being a parent is to teach children the difference between right and wrong. Children mainly learn this difference from watching their parents and from their friends rather than from their parents telling them what to do and what not to do.

### 15.5.1 Principles about discipline

- Children learn more from reward for good behaviour than from punishment for bad behaviour.
- The best rewards are signs of affection when the child has behaved well. A word of praise and a hug are often enough.
- Material rewards such as sweets or money should be small and given very soon after the good behaviour has occurred.
- When children are behaving badly, the best course is often to divert their attention to something they like to do.
- If they behave badly, children will often feel upset and less likely to repeat the behaviour if their parents simply tell them their behaviour is not acceptable.
- It is important for fathers and mothers to be consistent in their discipline. If one parent is more lax than the other parent, the child may try to play one parent off against the

other. Of course, mothers and fathers will behave differently to some degree. This will help children learn that family life and relationships are complicated.

- In some societies, it is common for parents to beat their children. In other countries it is illegal for parents to punish their children by hitting them. In general, hitting children for bad behaviour teaches them that people who are stronger and bigger can always get their own way. This is a negative lesson for children to learn. Parents who hit their children so hard that they leave marks on the skin may be accused of abuse. Children who are beaten are more likely to become anxious and aggressive later on in life.

## 15.6 Encouraging independence

Children need to become more responsible for their lives as they grow older. To encourage children to develop a level of independence that is appropriate for their age, parents should think of:

- consulting their children about decisions that will affect them – it is important too that parents take into account what their child says when they make a decision;
- encouraging them to do more and more for themselves – helping with the cooking, making their own bed, cleaning up after themselves – these are all tasks children should be expected to do, boys as much as girls.

Children should not, however, be expected to shoulder more responsibility than they can comfortably manage. It is not appropriate for children to be asked to decide, for example, whether their parents should separate or stay together, although if parents do separate, it is right that children should be asked where they would like to live, how often they would like to visit the other parent, etc.

## 15.7 Respecting the child as a person

Parents, teachers and friends are important influences on how a child's personality develops. Parents need to recognise and value the different personalities and talents their children have and not try to mould them into people they cannot be. A child who is easily upset may need to be more protected against stresses than one who is more robust. A child who is easily distracted may need a less stimulating environment than one who can concentrate well. The mother of a daughter who is shy may need to make greater efforts to help her child make friends than the mother of a very sociable girl.

## 15.8 Building self-esteem and confidence

Children are exposed to competition from an early age. This happens especially when they go to school. They will hear remarks such as 'My dad's better than your dad because he makes more money', 'My team's better than your team because we won the championship' or 'I'm better than you are because I got 84% on the test'.

This emphasis on competition is very strong in many societies. The health professional will sometimes find it hard or impossible to make parents feel differently. Parents should note the following.

- Success is less important than taking part and enjoying the experience.
- Children need to have targets that match ambition to ability. It is not sensible to put up unrealistic targets.

- Avoid humiliating children. For example, sarcastic comments are hurtful if a child does not do well. Use encouragement instead. Praise the child in the areas in which he does well, rather than shaming him where he does less well.
- Never link your love to achievement. Children need love however they achieve.
- When children are disappointed because they have not done well, let them express their feelings. But remind them how well they have done in the past.
- Give children the opportunity to meet challenges, for example by giving them tasks such as family games and household chores in which you know they can do well if they try.
- Do not hide your own failures. Let your children know of the times you have not done well. Children need to know their parents are not perfect.
- Set an example by treating competition in the way you would wish your children to do. Encourage enjoyment more than achievement.

Now you may like to prepare a talk you could give yourself to a group of parents in your own society on the needs of children. You could perhaps use the same headings, but with messages that are more in tune with the ideas in your own community.

# CHAPTER 16

# Mental health promotion

All health professionals know they have a duty not just to treat disease but to promote health. They do this partly by preventive measures such as vaccination and immunisation programmes. They also promote health by encouraging a healthy lifestyle, by giving advice on diet and exercise. As mental health problems contribute greatly to the total amount of ill health in the population, it makes sense for health professionals to be active in promoting mental health as well as encouraging good parenting (see Chapter 15).

## 16.1 Preventing intellectual disability

Intellectual disability has a permanent effect on an individual's quality of life. Although it cannot be entirely prevented, much can be done to help reduce the number of people who suffer from it. Health professionals have an important part to play.

### 16.1.1 Before the child is born

- Make sure mothers have enough to eat and get sufficient rest.
- Monitor the progress of the pregnancy regularly: refer to a gynaecologist if there is cause for concern about the health of the fetus or the mother.
- Discourage pregnancy before the age of 18.
- Discourage smoking, use of illicit drugs or drinking of alcohol in pregnancy, as it may harm the fetus.
- Treat as an emergency, high blood pressure or fits in pregnancy.
- Do not give pregnant mothers drugs or X-rays unless absolutely necessary.
- Advise pregnant women against carrying heavy loads or walking on slippery ground.
- Immunise mothers against measles and tetanus – do not let them come in contact with people with German measles, mumps or chicken pox.
- If there is a genetic counselling service available, refer all pregnant women over 40 as well as those with close relatives with intellectual disability.

### 16.1.2 At the time of childbirth

- Avoid premature childbirth if at all possible – if the mother enters labour too early, advise bed rest and refer.
- Ensure only skilled people conduct deliveries.
- If before delivery the baby is in an abnormal position, refer to a specialist.

### 16.1.3 After childbirth

- Ensure all babies are breastfed at least for the first 4 months of life; this prevents infection and ensures babies are adequately nourished.

- Ensure proper immunisations for diphtheria, polio, tetanus, tuberculosis, measles and whooping cough.
- Educate the family about proper nutrition.
- Ensure early control of any high fever with cold sponging and paracetamol.
- Treat repeated seizures with anticonvulsants.
- If possible, refer to a specialist all cases of jaundice and babies with breathing or serious feeding difficulties.
- Advise on parenting issues such as the importance of playing with children, talking to them and stimulating them, not abusing or neglecting them, limiting family size and ensuring a safe home with no access to drugs or poisons.

## 16.1.4 *Early intervention for babies at high risk*

- Babies may be at high risk because they have been born prematurely, with low birth weight, have had jaundice or meningitis, or have a genetic disorder such as Down syndrome. All babies need stimulation to develop well, but these babies are in special need of activities to promote their development.
- Principles of early intervention include:
    - finding out what the baby can and cannot do
    - deciding what the next steps for the baby should be
    - dividing each activity into small steps
    - choosing activities the parents can do to teach the child the relevant skills
    - encouraging the parents to repeat the activities each day. Children who are slow to develop need much more practice to master each skill.
- Some general guidelines for parents whose child is at risk of slow development include:
    - praise abundantly
    - talk a lot to the child about what they are doing
    - guide the child's movements with their hands, gradually decreasing support as the child is able to take on the activity on his own
    - use a mirror to increase the child's awareness of his body
    - teach by encouraging imitation
    - make learning fun by trying new things
    - involve other children in activities, as they can be the best teachers.
- Remember that children whose brain has been damaged during the pregnancy, or during or immediately after birth may not be capable of reaching the development of healthy children even with an immense amount of stimulation. All the same, early stimulation will give all children the best chance of reaching their potential.

## 16.2 Working with teachers

After the home, schools are the best places to promote mental health because:

- most children attend school at some time during their lives
- schools are often the strongest social and educational institutions available for intervention; schools have a profound influence on children, their families and the community
- young people's ability and motivation to stay in school, to learn and to make use of what they learn is affected by their mental well-being
- schools can act as a safety net, protecting children from dangers that affect their learning, development and psychosocial well-being

- schools, in addition to family, are crucial in building a child's self-esteem and sense of competence
- school mental health programmes are effective in improving learning and mental well-being and in reducing the stress on children with mental health disorders, thus achieving improvement in their conditions
- the school environment, by its very nature, can cause stress and strain on children – for example, stress due to examinations, low self-esteem in cases of failure, and depression in cases of bullying.

Teachers can run courses in the development of life skills. Children who have learned life skills to help them cope with stresses are less likely to develop behaviour and emotional problems. Life-skills courses need to be interactive, to be appropriate to the ages of the students and to engage their motivation. A life-skills course curriculum might cover the following subjects (Bharath *et al*, 2002):

- motivation for learning
- discipline
- nutrition
- health and hygiene
- relationships
- communication
- self-awareness
- sexuality
- social responsibility.

There are other ways in which schools can be involved. Teachers can promote mental health in students by creating a positive classroom environment in which teachers and students respect each other without shouting at or humiliating children.

Like parents, teachers need to encourage cooperation rather than competition. The emphasis on competition is deeply ingrained in many schools and it is not easy for health professionals to make a difference here. However, students should be taught to value participation as well as achievement. Cooperation brings with it a sense of belonging to a group. At least some of the work assignments given to children should involve the children interacting with each other. This will help build a sense of identity.

Teachers should avoiding humiliating students by making sarcastic comments. They should ensure that children feel safe by having classroom rules that are clearly displayed and respected. Reducing and, if possible, eliminating bullying in schools makes a major contribution to a feeling of safety at school (see Section 16.3 on anti-bullying programmes in schools).

The child's sense of purpose should be built on. This can be done by making sure teachers' expectations are realistic, that children are set achievable targets and that they are praised for good work, highlighting the best parts.

Helping students to be sympathetic and understanding to people with mental health problems can be achieved by:

- discussing people in the news who have revealed mental health problems such as depression (the probable stresses such people have experienced can be explained); or by
- arranging talks to students by people who themselves have mental health problems, so as to bring a human face to such problems. Discussing people who are in the news because of violent behaviour may also help. This can lead to discussion about ways in which people can resolve differences in non-violent ways.

In addition, students can be encouraged to get involved with the running of the school. This can be achieved by having a school council that discusses school rules. This will give students the opportunity, for example, to question school rules they think are unfair, make suggestions about the curriculum, and put forward ideas about new school events and celebrations. The existence of such a forum increases students' sense of self-worth.

Finally, schools should ensure that there is good communication at all levels within the organisation. This needs to begin at the top. Head teachers who keep their teaching staff up to date are more likely to have teachers who are good at communicating with each other and with their students.

## 16.2.1 Information about mental health problems and school

**Case 16.1**

Shanti is a 12-year-old girl who came with her mother to the clinic. Shanti had no wish to be present, but her mother made her show her wrists to the health professional. There were a number of cuts, mostly quite superficial, but one or two rather deep and poorly healed. It was obvious they had been self-inflicted. The health professional knew that Shanti was an unhappy, rather overweight girl who had never got over the fact that her father, to whom she had been close, had left home about 5 years earlier. She was an only child. She and her mother argued a lot, with Shanti blaming her mother for her father's absence. When the health professional asked Shanti why she had cut herself, Shanti said that a lot of the girls in her class at school cut themselves and then showed each other their cuts. It sounded as if they were proud of their behaviour. What should the health professional do?

There are very many reasons why it is helpful to children and parents if health professionals and teachers can communicate with each other freely, namely that it allows both parties to carry out their tasks effectively. Children can show behaviour and emotional problems either at home or at school, or in both places. Often, parents are surprised that children have problems in school because the child is fine at home. Similarly, teachers are sometimes surprised that a child has problems at home because there is nothing wrong at school. Children who are under stress at school may only show their emotions at home because they are frightened to show how they feel at school and vice versa. So, in order for a health professional to know what is going on, it is often important to understand what is happening in both environments.

Some mental health problems in school are epidemic in nature, i.e. children model or copy each other's behaviour. Examples of this are:

*   self-starvation or anorexia (see Section 9.3).
*   self-harming behaviour (see Section 9.4)
*   physical aggression (see Section 8.3)
*   cyberbullying (see Section 8.3.1).

There are numerous stresses that may be felt at school, including:

*   finding the work very hard
*   fear of failure in schoolwork
*   bullying (see Section 8.3.1)
*   dirty toilet facilities that children do not want to use.

Children with mental health problems, especially those with attention difficulties (ADHD), do much better if teachers recognise the problem. They can then modify their teaching approach to suit the child (see Section 8.2). For some physical and mental health problems such as epilepsy and diabetes, children may need to take medication in school. It is important that teachers are well informed about these children's needs.

Some school attendance problems, especially school refusal but also truancy, may benefit from the help of a health professional (see Sections 8.7). Schools can act as excellent bases for mental health promotion.

Note that the assessment and management of children who, for some reason, are not making good progress in their learning at school is dealt with in Chapters 4 and 5.

## 16.2.2 Communication between health professionals and teachers

Teachers and health professionals should partner parents to help children to live healthy lives and learn as well as possible. This means that, if at all possible, they need to find ways to communicate with each other. If they are able to communicate freely, this will help both groups of professionals to understand children's behaviour. This will make it easier for them to help.

The best methods of communication will depend on what is available. Face to face is best, but is time-consuming. On the other hand, mobile telephones and emails are all rapidly becoming more available as means of communication. Lack of time is probably the most frequently given reason for lack of communication, but remember that a short conversation that results in an explanation of a child's behaviour may save a lot of time in the long run.

Communication is sometimes made more difficult because teachers and health professionals have different ways of thinking about children. Health professionals mainly use a deficit model – 'What is wrong with this child?' – to restore children to health. Teachers mainly use a strengths model – 'We can build on what is right with this child' – to improve children's learning. So long as this is understood, useful conversations can take place.

Both teachers and health professionals are rightly concerned about confidentiality, especially not passing on information without the permission of parents. This is especially important when the information might be thought by the parents to be shameful. Teachers and health professionals need to be sensitive to this possibility. How they deal with it will depend on local rules and customs. Mostly, parents are happy for teachers and health professionals to communicate with each other about their children.

The actions teachers and health professionals take when given information by each other will depend on the nature of that information. For example, when there is a worrying epidemic of children copying each other in undesirable ways, teachers might:

- identify the child who is responsible for the other children's behaviour and remove him from the class temporarily
- talk to all the children affected, individually or as a group, to discuss how they might deal with their feelings in a different way
- talk to all the parents of the affected children, individually or as a group
- give the whole class the opportunity to learn about positive problem-solving techniques derived from CBT (see Section 2.3.1).

Schools are often the places where children learn to care for frail and vulnerable classmates. Learning to care for others may be one of the most important learning experiences children take away from their school days. It is also desirable to provide opportunities for helping others in the community through group activities.

Now make a list of the ways in which communication between the health professional who saw Shanti and her mother might be helpful.

# 16.3 Anti-bullying programmes in schools

**Case 16.2**

Rahul was a 10-year-old boy, small for his age and rather fat, whose father brought him to the clinic saying he just would not go to school. He had beaten Rahul many times to make him go, but it did not seem to make any difference. The health professional saw Rahul by himself for about 10 minutes. When asked why he would not go to school, Rahul said that he was frightened to go because two big boys beat him up in the break time. They teased him for being fat, called him 'fat lump' and asked him for money. When it turned out he did not have any money to give, they took him behind the toilets and hit him several times with their belts. This was the third time that the health professional had come across cases of bullying in the local school and she went to see the head teacher. The head teacher told her he knew there was bullying in the school, but what could he do? 'Boys will be boys', he said. What could the health professional do?

## *16.3.1 Information about bullying in schools*

Bullying occurs when a child is exposed to negative actions either by another child, usually bigger and stronger, or by a group of children. The negative actions may be hitting or teasing, threatening or calling names. Anxious, passive, physically weak children are most likely to be bullied.

Cyberbullying is a form of bullying that occurs when a child is exposed to mobile telephone texts, email or online social media messages that call the child names, humiliate, tease or threaten him. If the child who receives such messages is hurt or upset, the fact that the messages were only sent as a joke is not relevant. This is still cyberbullying.

Bullying is very common in many schools throughout the world. It is most common at 8–10 years. Boys are more involved in hitting and beating up other children; girls are more likely to use words to hurt other children, either face to face, electronically or through online forums.

Teachers often do not know about bullying. The more teachers there are at play times or break times, the less bullying there will be.

Being bullied is one of the most common reasons why children do not want to go to school. It is sometimes the main reason why children are depressed and, in a number of cases, it has actually driven children to attempt to kill themselves. Very occasionally, they have killed themselves.

Bullies are often aggressive children, not just to other children but to adults as well. They often show antisocial or other behaviour problems. Children who, at home, are poorly supervised and whose parents are themselves physically aggressive and deal with conflict by hitting out, are more likely to be bullies.

Bullying is more likely to occur in schools where it is tolerated and not taken seriously, and bullying by students is more likely to occur when there is bullying of teachers in the staff room – for example, inexperienced teachers may be humiliated by more senior teachers. This creates a culture of bullying in the school.

## 16.3.2 What can be done about bullying in schools?

Note that some of the suggestions in this section may not be suitable for schools in some societies. Health professionals need to be sensitive to the culture of the schools attended by their patients.

Although individual children who are being bullied need understanding and help, action on bullying can only be effective if it is taken by teachers and the school authorities. The following are measures that have been successfully taken to reduce or even remove bullying in schools.

### School authorities

The school authority needs to make it clear to the head teacher that they expect her school to take measures to reduce bullying and that this is as much part of her job as producing good academic results. School authorities should not, however, bully head teachers by threatening them if they do not get good results. Instead, they need to provide encouragement and support to head teachers to enable them to do a better job.

### Head teachers

- Nurture their teaching staff, especially the weaker members, and avoid making them feel inadequate.
- Make sure it is understood by all teachers and students that bullying is not to be tolerated.
- Make sure that her teachers understand that humiliating children in the classroom is not acceptable behaviour, and help them to find other ways to encourage weaker students.
- Make sure that playgrounds are well supervised at break and play times, and regular checks are made on places that are difficult to supervise, such as in and behind the lavatories.
- Be easily available to parents who wish to talk about their children being bullied.
- Arrange supervised meetings between parents of children who are bullied and parents of children who are bullying them.
- Prohibit the use of mobile telephones in school.

### Class teachers

- Introduce as much cooperative learning or small group work as possible. This means that children are expected to work together in pairs or small groups at least some of the time. Such experience reduces the likelihood that children will be aggressive to each other because they will depend on each other.
- Be available to parents who wish to talk about their child being bullied.
- Have class rules about bullying, including cyberbullying by text or email messaging.
- Set up a system so that children can report episodes of bullying anonymously. One way of doing this is to have a box into which students can drop notes without anyone knowing they have done this.
- Make sure that mobile telephones are not used in the classroom or at other times while children are in school.
- Praise the class when no bullying has occurred for some time. This should occur after every break time if bullying is frequent, less often otherwise.

- Ensure that when bullying is identified, the bully is talked to very seriously about his behaviour and the effect it is having. Punishment may need to take place but should not involve any sort of public humiliation.
- Be prepared to talk to parents of children who are bullies as well as parents of children who are bullied about what is happening.

**Parents**

- Make sure their children tell them if they are being bullied.
- Be prepared to tell the head teacher or class teacher if their child is being bullied.
- Cooperate with the school in all the measures the school is taking to reduce bullying, especially if their child is involved in bullying.

Now write down how the health professional who saw Rahul and his father might approach the head teacher or class teacher.

# 16.4 Social networking

**Case 16.3**

Shreya, a 12-year-old girl, was brought by her angry mother to the health professional. Her mother said that Shreya had met a boy on the internet and 'fallen in love' with him. Now she wanted to go and visit him in a town about 40 miles away. Nothing that her mother could say would change her mind. Her mother suspected that, although the boy she was writing to said he was 16 years old, he was probably much older and might well be a married man. She had seen some of the messages the two had sent to each other. They were very intimate and not at all appropriate, the mother felt, for a girl of Shreya's age. There was no way she was going to let Shreya go off to meet this man. But Shreya was threatening to run away. What should the health professional advise?

## 16.4.1 Information on social networking

Our mental well-being is affected by things that we do regularly and, as social beings, a healthy social life is an important aspect of this. In many parts of the world, including LAMI countries, a new way in which young people communicate with each other and regularly spend their time is by social networking. Children as young as those in primary school are spending a significant time on the internet and other social media.

Social networking is an important aspect of young people's lives today. It has both negative and positive impacts, depending on a variety of factors. Positive aspects of social networking include the ability to connect with other people regardless of distance, time or physical circumstances. Negative impacts are often more difficult to recognise. The greatest concerns for young people who overuse social networking are social isolation, bullying and depression. Young people, particularly those in their teens, are prone to poor self-esteem and depression. They are also more sensitive about how other people think of them. Young people who are desperate for friendship make poor choices and this is easier to do on the internet. They can readily become victims of bullying and emotional abuse.

Some young people are heavy users of the internet, developing what is, in fact, an internet addiction. This can be said to exist when such activity is pursued at the expense of any other activity. Young people who are so taken up with the social media may not take part at all in any 'offline' activities. These children are more likely to have depression and be lonely.

## 16.4.2 Assessment of possible overuse of the internet

The following signs are helpful in recognising children who are at risk.

- Spending less time engaged in talking, sharing or communicating with others.
- Difficulties in attention and concentration and lack of focus in schoolwork or other activities of daily living.
- Lack of interest in one-to-one or group relationships; making the internet more important than activities with family and friends.
- Lack of interest and engagement in any 'offline' social activities; feels a constant urge to check status updates and communicate online.
- Frustration, agitation and other withdrawal symptoms (fidgeting, aggression, etc.) when unable to engage in online or social media related activities.

In order to avoid these problems, parents need to encourage their children to be involved in a variety of activities, including face-to-face social engagements and outdoor activities.

Although these problems occur and indeed are widespread, there are very positive aspects in the use of new technology. Moderation in the time spent and recognising the dangers of online relationships and cyberbullying (see Section 8.3.1) are critical.

# CHAPTER 17

# Medication

This chapter provides general information on medication and its use. Please see other sections in this manual for additional information relating to the use of medication in specific mental health conditions.

1. Medication should only be used when it has been possible to make a diagnosis of a mental disorder. The emotional and behaviour problems shown by many children do not usually fit into any diagnostic category. Children with these problems may well need therapeutic interventions, especially listening and talking treatments. However, medication should be used for cases where a diagnosis has been made and there are clear treatment goals.

2. Not all health professionals are allowed to prescribe medication. Each country has its own regulations. Some of the medications mentioned in Appendix 2 have a lot of evidence to say that they are useful (e.g. stimulants for ADHD). Many other medications do not have such evidence. For detailed accounts of the medication, please see suggested reading (p. 197). When in doubt before (or even after) starting the medication, refer to or communicate with an expert with experience in using medication in children.

3. The general dictum to follow while giving medication to children with mental disorders is: start low, go slow. Allow time for adequate trial before deciding to change the medication, especially in chronic disorders (e.g. it may take 4–8 weeks for a child with depression or schizophrenia to respond to the medication). Where possible, change one medication at a time.

4. All types of medication have side-effects. It is important to warn parents about these when you first prescribe them. If possible, get the mother to tell you before the child starts medication whether the child is showing any of these already. Then, if a side-effect is later reported, you will be able to tell whether the child was already showing this problem before he began to take the medication.

5. Many parents are worried about their children being given tablets to alter their mind or behaviour. You will need to discuss their worries, and if they have strong negative feelings, you may not be able to prescribe the medication. It may be helpful to say things like 'I think you are quite right to worry about X going on to tablets. I would worry too. But I don't often prescribe medication for children and I have to say that if this were my child, I would consider a trial of medication'.

6. Medication should never be given without first listening and talking to both the child and the parents. With children on medication it is really important to continue to listen to and talk with parents and the children about the stresses in their lives and how these can be reduced.

7. Choice of treatment will depend on the nature of the problem and on the resources available to the health professional. Some form of intervention combining medication

with a talking treatment may be the best intervention if this can be achieved. For example, moderate to severe depression or obsessive–compulsive disorder responds better to a combination of medication and CBT. You need to bear in mind how willing the patient and family are likely to be in taking the medication, and whether they can afford to buy the medication or pay for the transport to come to the centre. Try not to suggest a treatment if you think the family will not be able to cooperate. If you prescribe medication, for example, and the child does not take it, you may only have succeeded in giving the child another reason for feeling he has failed.

8    Do find out before you start treatment which interventions have already been tried. Asking the parent questions such as 'I wonder what you've already tried to help with this problem' may save you a lot of time.

9    One would do well to ask the parent 'So how have you understood your child's problem?' or 'What do your family elders think this is due to?', or if they have seen someone already for the problem 'What did the previous doctor say?' Checking with the parent on their own views and understanding of the problem can sometimes help you to be more effective.

10   Treatments are much more likely to work if the parents and child like and have confidence in the health professional who is prescribing them. As a busy health professional you will only have limited time to get to know the families you treat. Whatever you can do to inspire confidence in your patients will make both listening and talking treatments and medication more likely to work. Find out whether the head of the family can come to one of the visits, so that a connection is established with the person who takes decisions.

11   It is really important to make sure you find out what the effects of your treatment have been. Monitoring outcomes in the target symptoms and in more than one setting is important. It will help you to decide what to do in the future not just with the child you are currently treating but with other children that you will see in the future.

# References and suggested reading

## References

Bharath, S., Kishore Kumar, K. V. & Vranda, M. N. (2002) *Activity Manual for the Teachers on Health Promotion using Life Skills Approach (Eighth Standard)*. Department of Psychiatry, National Institute of Mental Health and Neuro Sciences, India.

Bryanne, B. & Eapen, V. (2012) The infant with special meaning. In *Contemporary Approaches to Child and Adolescent Mental Health: Volume 1, Infancy and Childhood* (eds L. Newman & S. Mares), pp. 10–25. IP Communications.

Clinical Center (2006) *Patient Information Publications: Talking to Children about Death*. National Institutes of Health.

Gershoff, E. T., Grogan-Kaylor, A., Lansford, J. E., *et al* (2010) Parent discipline practices in an international sample: associations with child behaviors and moderation by perceived normativeness. *Child Development*, **81**, 487–502.

Giel, R., de Arango, M. V., Climent, C. E., *et al* (1981) Childhood mental disorders in primary health care: results of observations in four developing countries. *Pediatrics*, **68**, 677–683.

Patel, V. (2003) *Where There Is No Psychiatrist: A Mental Health Care Manual*. Gaskell.

Turk, J., Graham, P. & Verhulst, F. C. (2007) *Child and Adolescent Psychiatry: A Developmental Approach* (4th edn). Oxford University Press.

## Suggested reading

Barkley, R. A. & Benton, C. M. (1998) *Your Defiant Child*. Guilford Press.

Centers for Disease Control and Prevention (2001) Data table of BMI-for-age charts. CDC (http://www.cdc.gov/growthcharts/html_charts/bmiagerev.htm).

Eapen, V., Kulhara, P. & Raguram, R. (2012) *Essentials of Psychiatry* (2nd edn). Paras Publishing.

Girimaji, S. R. (1998) *Counsellors Manual for Family Intervention in Mental Retardation*. Indican Council of Medical Research, National Institute of Mental Health and Neuro Sciences.

Seshadri, S., Saksena, S. & Saldanha, S. (2008) *On Track: A Series on Life Skills and Personal Safety. Book 1 to 7 (Classes 3 to 9)*. Macmillan India.

Stallard, P. (2005) *A Clinician's Guide to Think Good–Feel Good: Using CBT with Children and Young People*. John Wiley.

Woods, D. W. (2008) *Managing Tourette Syndrome: A Behavioral Intervention for Children and Adults. Therapist Guide* (eBook). Oxford University Press.

World Health Organization (2001) *Counselling Skills Training in Adolescent Sexuality and Reproductive Health: A Facilitator's Guide (WHO/ADH/93)* (updated version). WHO.

World Health Organization (2012) Global database on body mass index: an interactive surveillance tool for monitoring nutrition transition. WHO (http://apps.who.int/bmi/index.jsp).

World Health Organization (2012) The WHO Child Growth Standards. WHO (http://www.who.int/childgrowth/standards/en/).

# Appendix 1

## My Star Chart

Name: ..............................................................................................................................

| | | | | | |
|---|---|---|---|---|---|
| Monday | ☆ | ☆ | ☆ | ☆ | ☆ |
| Tuesday | ☆ | ☆ | ☆ | ☆ | ☆ |
| Wednesday | ☆ | ☆ | ☆ | ☆ | ☆ |
| Thursday | ☆ | ☆ | ☆ | ☆ | ☆ |
| Friday | ☆ | ☆ | ☆ | ☆ | ☆ |
| Saturday | ☆ | ☆ | ☆ | ☆ | ☆ |
| Sunday | ☆ | ☆ | ☆ | ☆ | ☆ |

# Appendix 2: Guide to medication for use in childhood mental disorders

Table A1 Medications commonly used in childhood mental disorders

| Disorder | Medication | How to use | Important side-effects | Points to remember |
|---|---|---|---|---|
| Attention-deficit hyperactivity disorder (ADHD) | **First line**<br>*Stimulants*<br>1. Methylphenidate<br>  i. short acting (3–4h)<br>  ii. long acting (8–12h)<br>2. Dexamphetamine (3–6h duration of action)<br>Stimulants are Schedule III drugs – availability varies between countries. Country-specific rules need to be followed when prescribing<br>Individual responsiveness (which may be genetically determined) varies<br><br>**Second line**<br>*Non-stimulants*<br>1. Atomoxetine<br>2. Clonidine | **Stimulants**<br>*Short-acting methylphenidate*<br>0.3–0.5 mg/kg/dose<br>Start at 5 mg OD/BD and increase by 5–10 mg weekly increments to a maximum dose of 1 mg/kg/day or 60 mg/day<br>Can be given up to 2–3 doses per day – last dose should not be given after 16:00–17:00 h<br>Start at 2.5–5.0 mg, increase weekly (up-titration)<br><br>*Long-acting methylphenidate*<br>0.5–2.0 mg/kg OD dose<br>Maximum 60 mg/day<br><br>*Dexamphetamine*<br>Start at 2.5 mg OD/BD and increase by 2.5–5 mg weekly increments to a maximum of 0.5 mg/kg/day or 40 mg/day<br><br>**Non-stimulants**<br>*Atomoxetine*<br>Initiate at 0.5 mg/kg/day and increase every week to a target of 1.2 mg/kg<br>Maximum daily dose: body weight <70 kg, 80 mg/day; body weight >70 kg, 100 mg/day<br>OD/BD dosing; can be given in the evening<br><br>*Clonidine*<br>3–7 μg/kg/day, maximum dose 0.3 mg<br>Start with 25–50 μg and increase by 25 μg increments every 3–4 days<br>Wait for 4 weeks for full therapeutic response<br>OD at bedtime or BD dosing<br><br>**General**<br>Trial of discontinuation by tapering can be given after 1–2 years of adequate symptom control | **Stimulants**<br>Loss of appetite, ↓ sleep, irritability/instability/moodiness, alter pulse rate and blood pressure, may slow down growth (need to monitor weight, height, growth, blood pressure and pulse)<br>Lowers seizure threshold – should be used with adequate precaution in children with seizures and only after the seizures are well controlled<br><br>**Non-stimulants**<br>*Atomoxetine*<br>↓ appetite, nausea, vomiting, ↓ sleep or tiredness, dry mouth<br><br>*Clonidine*<br>Sedation, dizziness, dry mouth<br>At times, paradoxical worsening of symptoms and mood may be seen<br>Monitor blood pressure as it is an antihypertensive and may lower blood pressure (rare) | **Stimulants**<br>Tics may be precipitated or worsened in some children<br>Ask about personal or family history of tics, seizures or heart disease<br>Not to give the medicine after 16:00–17:00 h, otherwise it may disturb sleep<br>Supervised dosing in adolescents may also be needed in school to prevent inappropriate use and potential distribution to peers<br><br>**Non-stimulants**<br>*Atomoxetine*<br>Avoid in case of jaundice/liver disease (pre-existing or emergent)<br>Keep a watch for suicidal thinking that can emerge with this medication<br><br>*Clonidine*<br>Not to stop suddenly due to risk of rebound severe hypertension<br>Useful in treating tics with or without ADHD as it is beneficial for both conditions, improves sleep |
| Depression | Psychotherapy should be considered before drugs<br><br>***First line (SSRIs)***<br>Fluoxetine<br><br>***Second line (SSRIs)***<br>Sertraline<br>Citalopram<br>Escitalopram | **SSRIs**<br>1. Start low (fluoxetine 5–10 mg, sertraline 12.5 mg, citalopram/escitalopram 2.5 mg, TCAs 10–25 mg)<br>2. Increase dose slowly to minimise the risk of treatment-emergent agitation<br>3. At least weekly follow up in the early stages of treatment<br>4. In early phase of treatment, monitor for suicidality or agitation | **SSRIs**<br>↓ appetite, nausea, headache, insomnia, delayed ejaculation, ↓ sexual desire<br>Stop in case of agitation or undue cheerfulness/excitement with sleep disturbance<br>Monitor for suicidality that can occur with the use of SSRIs | Antidepressants need to be added if there is little or no response to 4–6 weeks of psychotherapy, or if depression is moderate to severe, or psychotherapy is simply not available<br>SSRIs have mostly replaced TCAs for depression in children<br>Adolescents can be expected to respond better to antidepressants than younger children |

*Continued*

Table A1 Medications commonly used in childhood mental disorders

| Disorder | Medication | How to use | Important side-effects | Points to remember |
|---|---|---|---|---|
| Depression (cont.) | **Third line (TCAs)** Imipramine Amitriptyline **Avoid** Paroxetine and venlafaxine | 5. Maximum daily dose: fluoxetine 20–40 mg, sertraline 100–200 mg, citalopram/escitalopram 10–20 mg, TCAs 150 mg 6. Should be continued for at least 1 year of symptom-free period | **TCAs** Sedation, weight gain, dry mouth, constipation May also cause urinary retention, glaucoma, changes in heart rhythm (baseline and on-treatment ECG are needed) | |
| Obsessive–compulsive disorder | **First line (SSRIs)** Sertraline Fluoxetine Fluvoxamine Citalopram Escitalopram **Second line (TCA)** Clomipramine | 1. Start low (sertraline 12.5 mg, fluoxetine 5–10 mg, fluvoxamine 25 mg, citalopram/escitalopram 2.5–5 mg, clomipramine 10–25 mg) 2. Increase dose slowly to minimise the risk of treatment emergent agitation 3. At least weekly follow up in the early stages of treatment 4. In early phase of treatment, monitor for suicidality or agitation 5. Maximum daily dose: sertraline 150–250 mg, fluoxetine 40–60 mg, fluvoxamine 150–250 mg, clomipramine 150 mg 6. Should be continued for 6 months to 1 year of symptom-free period. If reduction of dose causes relapse, may need to continue indefinitely. | **SSRIs** ↓ appetite, nausea, headache, insomnia, delayed ejaculation, ↓ sexual desire Stop in case of agitation or undue cheerfulness/excitement with sleep disturbance Monitor for suicidality that can occur with the use of SSRIs **TCAs** Sedation, weight gain, dry mouth, constipation May also cause urinary retention, glaucoma, changes in heart rhythm (baseline and on-treatment ECG are needed) | All children and adolescents with obsessive–compulsive disorder should be offered CBT, even if they are on medication |
| Anxiety disorders (generalised anxiety disorder, separation anxiety, specific phobias, social phobia, PTSD) | Psychotherapy should be considered before drugs **Acute and short-term control (2–4 weeks)** Benzodiazepines (lorazepam, clonazepam, alprazolam, diazepam) **Long-term management** SSRIs Fluoxetine (drug of choice) Fluvoxamine Sertraline **Anxiolytic** Buspirone (mainly as an add-on agent) **Avoid** TCAs | **Benzodiazepines** Daily dose ranges: lorazepam 0.5–4 mg in up to 4 divided doses; clonazepam 0.25–2.0 mg in up to 3 divided doses; diazepam 2.5–20.0 mg in up to 3 divided doses; alprazolam 0.125–1.0 mg in up to 3 divided doses Use lowest possible effective dose for shortest possible time and then taper off **SSRIs** *Fluoxetine* Start with 2.5 mg in the morning and increase by 2.5 mg every week up to 10–20 mg/day (OD dose) *Fluvoxamine* Start with 25 mg and increase weekly by 25 mg up to 100–125 mg/day (night doses or BD doses with larger dose at night) | **Benzodiazepines** Sedation, dizziness Forgetfulness, ataxia (less common at lower doses) Can cause dependence, paradoxical worsening or excitation **SSRIs** ↓ appetite, nausea, headache, insomnia, delayed ejaculation, ↓ sexual desire Stop in case of agitation or undue cheerfulness/excitement with sleep disturbance Monitor for suicidality that can occur with the use of SSRIs **Anxiolytic (buspirone)** Sedation, dizziness Can occasionally cause disinhibition and worsen aggression (less common than in benzodiazepines) | CBT is usually the recommended first-line treatment. If anxiety is severe or disabling and CBT is unavailable or has failed, use of medication should be considered Combination of CBT and SSRI is superior to both therapies alone Alprazolam and mouth-dissolving clonazepam are often used to curb a panic attack (immediate action) Children are more likely to develop excitation/disinhibition with benzodiazepines than adults. Need to monitor for the same Rapid reduction of benzodiazepines can precipitate seizures in vulnerable children (past/personal/family history of seizure disorder needs to be known) Buspirone does not cause dependence or withdrawal |

Continued

Table A1 Medications commonly used in childhood mental disorders

| Disorder | Medication | How to use | Important side-effects | Points to remember |
|---|---|---|---|---|
| Anxiety (cont.) | | *Sertraline*<br>Start with 12.5 mg morning and increase every week by 12.5–25 mg up to 100–125 mg/day (OD dose)<br>Continue for at least 1 year of symptom-free period<br><br>***Anxiolytic (buspirone)***<br>Start with 2.5 mg 2–3 times a day<br>Maximum dose 15–20 mg/day | | |
| Psychosis (early-onset schizophrenia, acute psychosis) | **SGAs**<br>Risperidone<br>Olanzapine<br>Quetiapine<br>Aripiprazole<br>Amisulpride<br>Clozapine (most effective in treatment-resistant cases)<br><br>*Avoid*<br>Ziprasidone (can cause cardiac arrhythmia)<br><br>**FGAs**<br>Haloperidol<br>Chlorpromazine<br>Sulpiride | Use the lowest effective dose<br>For acute psychosis, mania with psychotic symptoms and psychotic depression, antipsychotics can be tapered off after at least 6 months of symptom-free period<br>For schizophrenia, a trial of discontinuation can be given by gradually tapering after 6 months of symptom-free period<br>High rates of relapse are known and may require to continue indefinitely<br><br>**SGAs**<br>*Risperidone*<br>Start with 0.25–0.5 mg BD, maximum dose 4–6 mg/day<br><br>*Olanzapine*<br>Start with 2.5 mg night or BD dose, maximum dose 15–20 mg/day<br><br>*Quetiapine*<br>Start with 25 mg BD, maximum dose 400–800 mg/day<br><br>*Aripiprazole*<br>Start with 2 mg OD, maximum dose 10 mg/day<br><br>*Sulpiride/amisulpride*<br>Start with 25–50 mg BD, maximum dose 400–800 mg/day<br><br>*Clozapine*<br>Start with 12.5 mg BD, weekly increase 25 mg/day, maximum dose 300–350 mg/day<br><br>*Haloperidol*<br>Start with 0.5 mg, maximum dose 15–20 mg/day BD/TID<br><br>*Chlorpromazine*<br>Start with 25 mg BD, maximum dose 400 mg/day | **SGAs**<br>May cause weight gain, sedation, and metabolic abnormalities including obesity, insulin resistance, type 2 diabetes and metabolic syndrome<br>Seizures, agranulocytosis, myocarditis (rare), hypersalivation with clozapine<br><br>**FGAs**<br>Sedation, constipation, extrapyramidal or Parkinsonism-like symptoms with tremor and rigidity, acute muscle spasms or dystonia, akathesia, and tardive dyskinesia in long-term use<br>Weight gain in some children on chlorpromazine | Mostly, FGAs have been replaced by SGAs<br><br>***Other uses of antipsychotics***<br>Mania in bipolar disorder, psychotic depression, impulsive/aggressive behaviours<br>Haloperidol (0.5–3 mg/day) and risperidone (0.25–2.0 mg/day) in tics and Tourette syndrome<br>Risperidone is particularly useful in autism for disruptive behaviours and aggression<br>Patients on SGAs need monitoring for BMI and metabolic parameters<br>Patients on olanzapine will need monitoring for liver function tests in addition to weight gain and type 2 diabetes<br>Patients on clozapine will need monitoring for blood count and baseline ECG and EEG |

*Continued*

Table A1 Medications commonly used in childhood mental disorders

| Disorder | Medication | How to use | Important side-effects | Points to remember |
|---|---|---|---|---|
| Bipolar disorder | **First-line mood stabilisers**<br>Lithium<br>Valproic acid (sodium valproate, divalproex)<br><br>**Second-line mood stabilisers**<br>Carbamazepine<br>Lamotrigine<br><br>**Third-line/add-on mood stabilisers**<br>Oxcarbazepine<br>Topiramate<br><br>**Antipsychotics with mood-stabilising/anti-manic effects**<br>Risperidone<br>Olanzapine<br>Aripiprazole | Mood stabilisers are mostly needed to continue indefinitely. In first episode of mania, a mood stabiliser can be started if euphoria/irritability is not settling within 1–2 weeks of antipsychotic (SGA) treatment or the risk of another episode is high (severe symptoms, family history of bipolar disorder)<br><br>*Lithium*<br>Start with 300–450 mg/day in 2–3 divided doses and titrate upwards according to blood levels (desired blood level 0.8–1.2 mEq/l)<br><br>*Valproic acid*<br>20–30 mg/kg/day in 2–3 divided doses<br><br>*Carbamazepine*<br>10–20 mg/kg/day in 2–3 divided doses<br><br>*Lamotrigine*<br>Start with 12.5 mg/day. Weekly increase by 12.5 mg. Administer BD dose. Maximum dose 100–200 mg/day<br><br>*Oxcarbazepine*<br>Start with 8–10 mg/kg in two divided doses<br><br>*Topiramate*<br>Maximum dose 75–100 mg/day<br><br>*Risperidone*<br>Start with 0.25–0.5 mg BD, maximum dose 4–6 mg/day<br><br>*Olanzapine*<br>Start with 2.5 mg night or BD dose, maximum dose 15–20 mg/day<br><br>*Aripiprazole*<br>Start with 2 mg OD, maximum dose of 10 mg/day | *Lithium*<br>Excessive thirst, frequent urination, acne, weight gain, tremors<br><br>*Valproic acid*<br>Sedation, tremor, weight gain, gastrointestinal symptoms, hair loss, can cause liver function abnormality and polycystic ovarian disease<br><br>*Carbamazepine*<br>Dizziness, incoordination, skin rash (at times severe, e.g. Stevens–Johnson syndrome), can cause ↓ white blood cells<br><br>*Lamotrigine*<br>Skin rash needs to be monitored for the first 8 weeks. May cause Stevens–Johnson syndrome.<br><br>*Topiramate*<br>Dizziness, renal stones, metabolic acidosis, reduced appetite, recent memory difficulties, word retrieving difficulties | Except lithium, the other mood stabilisers are also used as anticonvulsants<br>Monotherapy and starting doses at the lower end of the therapeutic range should be by default<br>Lithium: monitoring needed for blood level, thyroid and renal function; monitor for signs of toxicity, especially in dry weather, dehydration<br>Lithium and lamotrigine are useful in the depressive phase of bipolar disorder<br>Valproic acid, carbamazepine and lithium can be used in episodic aggression/rage attacks/aggression with severe mood dysregulation episodes<br>Topiramate can be added on when weight control or seizure control is needed. Can cause behavioural problems. |
| Insomnia | *First line*<br>Melatonin<br><br>*Second line*<br>Benzodiazepines<br>Lorazepam<br>Clonazepam<br><br>*Non-benzodiazepine hypnotic*<br>Zolpidem | *Melatonin*<br>1.5–3.0 mg/night for sleep onset delay; 3–6 mg/night as a hypnotic<br><br>*Lorazepam*<br>Start with 0.05 mg/kg (maximum 2 mg/dose) and can be repeated every 4–8 h<br><br>*Clonazepam*<br>Start with 0.01 and 0.03 mg/kg/day but do not exceed 0.05 mg/kg/day given in 2–3 divided doses<br><br>*Zolpidem*<br>6.25–12.5 mg/night; short-term use only (2–4 weeks) | *Melatonin*<br>Can cause headache, irritability, nausea, palpitation, itching<br>May worsen seizures/asthma<br><br>*Zolpidem*<br>Can cause dizziness, headache and, rarely, excitation/disinhibition | Melatonin is used in autism, ADHD and depression when children have sleep difficulties<br>Zolpidem is more expensive than benzodiazepines. It helps in reducing night-time awakenings, has fewer side-effects and causes less dependence than benzodiazepines. |

*Continued*

193

Table A1 Medications commonly used in childhood mental disorders

| Disorder | Medication | How to use | Important side-effects | Points to remember |
|---|---|---|---|---|
| Extrapyramidal side-effects caused by antipsychotic drugs | **Anticholinergic drugs**<br>Benztropine<br>Trihexyphenidyl (as anti-Parkinsonian agent in adolescents) | **Benztropine**<br>0.02–0.05 mg/kg/dose OD/BD to a maximum dose of 0.1 mg/kg or 2–4 mg<br>(If oral dose is not possible, the intramuscular or intravenous dose is 0.02 mg/kg stat; may repeat in 15 minutes)<br><br>**Trihexyphenidyl**<br>1-2mg/dose based on need<br>Maximum dose of 4–6mg/day in divided doses | **Benztropine**<br>Can cause dry mouth, blurred vision, constipation, urinary retention, tachycardia, anorexia, drowsiness, disorientation<br><br>**Trihexyphenidyl**<br>Same side-effects as above | Benztropine should not be used in children under 3 years. It may decrease sweating and the body's ability to cool itself. The child will need to take care when outside in hot weather and will need to drink extra fluids. |

BD, twice daily; BMI, body mass index; CBT, cognitive–behavioural therapy; ECG, electrocardiogram; EEG electroencephalogram; FGA, first-generation antipsychotic; OD, once daily; PTSD, post-traumatic stress disorder; SGA, second-generation antipsychotic; SSRI, selective serotonin reuptake inhibitor; TCA, tricyclic antidepressant; TID, three times daily.

# Index

Compiled by Linda English

Printed in the United States
by Baker & Taylor Publisher Services